THE S.

THE
SLEEP
technique

Simple secrets for a deep,
restorative night's sleep

ANTHEA COURTENAY

Thorsons
An Imprint of HarperCollins*Publishers*

Thorsons
An Imprint of HarperCollins*Publishers*
77–85 Fulham Palace Road
Hammersmith, London w6 8jb

Published by Thorsons 1999

10 9 8 7 6 5 4 3 2

A catalogue record for this book
is available from the British Library

ISBN 0 7225 3793 X

Printed in Great Britain by
Woolnough Bookbinding Ltd,
Irthlingborough, Northamptonshire

Contents

Introduction VII

1. What is sleep? 1
2. Insomnia 11
3. Seeking the cause 18
4. The habit of insomnia 25
5. Restoring the balance 35
6. The churning mind 44
7. Your sleep and other people 53
8. A healthy environment 61
9. Balancing your lifestyle 66
10. A change of pace 79
11. Food and other habits 94
12. Bedtime 107
13. How natural therapies can help 122
14. The therapies 128

Introduction

A good, undisturbed night's sleep is one of the most enjoyable and totally natural pleasures available to us, yet for many people sleep is hard to come by. This in turn affects the quality of their waking life.

Sleep and dreams are as much a part of life as being busy and active; they unwind the body and mind, restoring our energies to face the next day. Yet how many people regularly wake feeling really refreshed? It has been estimated that at some time half the British population will be affected by insomnia. And many people, while not long-term insomniacs, experience times when the quality of their sleep is not all it could be.

Whether you suffer from full-blown insomnia or poor sleeping patterns, this book is for you. *The Sleep Technique* will help you to break out of poor sleep habits and bring your whole life into balance. Find out how natural medicine such as herbalism and aromatherapy can help, as well as self-help methods such as exercise, relaxation and adopting a change of lifestyle. Use this positive, easy-to-follow guide and your sleep problems will be a thing of the past.

CHAPTER I

What is sleep?

It is an extraordinary fact that something that occupies up to a third of our lives is still a mystery. Of course, we all know that sleep gives us rest: without it we feel tired and irritable and don't function as well as we'd like. Since 1952, sleep research laboratories attached to universities have been studying sleep patterns, with the help of human guinea-pigs. They have made numerous investigations not just into how we sleep but *why*, and no one has yet come up with a complete answer.

If you are beset by insomnia, you might wonder what use such investigations are. Whatever sleep is *for*, you know you need it and feel rotten without it. But the results of many of these investigations can offer some reassurance to the non-sleeper. They have, for instance, blown away the myth that everyone needs eight hours a night. Some of them suggest that most of us could get by

on less sleep than we have without coming to harm.
And some have come up with ideas for improving sleep.

In sleep the brain goes through four main stages,
each characterized by different types of brainwave – the
electrical impulses emitted by the brain.

SLEEP STATES

Stage 1: This first stage, the lightest, is the transition from
wakefulness to drowsiness; as we enter it our muscles
relax, the blood pressure drops, and the heart rate and
digestion slow down. The brain begins to produce
hormones such as serotonin and melatonin which are
associated with sleep and sleepiness (whether they actually
cause sleep is under debate).

At the same time, there is an increase in alpha waves,
brainwaves of 7–14 cycles per second, which are typical
of relaxed wakefulness; alpha waves also appear in
people who are meditating, or under hypnosis. This

stage lasts between one and ten minutes in the normal sleeper; although we return to it at intervals during the night, it usually occupies only about 5 per cent of our sleep.

Stage 2: This stage starts quite soon after falling asleep and occupies about 45 per cent of human sleep. It contains a mixture of deeper, slower brainwaves: theta brainwaves (3.5–7.5 cycles per second) typical of drowsiness and light sleep, and slow delta waves (under 3.5 cycles per second), during which we are really unconscious.

Stage 3: which occupies only about 7 per cent of sleep in young adults, is another transition phase to deeper sleep; as delta wave activity increases, we are taken fairly rapidly to Stage 4.

Stage 4: is the deepest form of sleep, with delta brainwaves predominating; it makes us about 13 per cent of sleep in the young adult. We stay in Stage 4 for quite long periods before surfacing again to REM and Stage 1 several times during the night.

REM Sleep: Rapid Eye Movement sleep is so called because the sleeper's eyes move, indicating that they are dreaming. It occurs during Stage 1 sleep, and increases in quantity later on in the night. It has now been found that we also dream during deeper stages of sleep.

It used to be thought that REM sleep was the part of sleep essential to us; it was believed that these stages were needed for brain rest, and that people deprived of them would develop psychosis. This last has been disproved, though deprivation of REM sleep does produce irritability and difficulties in concentration, and affects the ability to retain information learned the day before. People totally deprived of REM for more than three days have started having waking dreams, in the form of hallucinations. Others have been found to become less inhibited and conscientious.

CORE SLEEP

In his book, *Why We Sleep* (OUP, 1988), sleep research expert Dr Jim Horne proposes that the really essential part of sleep consists of Stages 3 and 4, which he calls collectively Slow Wave Sleep (SWS). During these stages the brain is in what he calls an 'off-line' state: it is the only time during which this hard-working organ is totally at rest. SWS occurs largely during the first three cycles, that is, during the first half of a night's sleep.

When people are deprived of sleep by staying up all night, it has been found that they don't need to catch up with all the sleep they've lost. They recover no extra light sleep, and only a fraction of REM sleep. But they do recover all the lost deep sleep, which suggests that that is the sleep that is really essential.

In people who naturally need less sleep than the average, the same pattern is followed during the first few hours as in average sleepers. Although these people sleep for fewer hours, says Dr Horne, they are getting the essential Slow Wave Sleep: 'It is as though these short sleepers have somehow done away with what seems to be the flexible non-restorative sleep – the latter hours of sleep.'

His conclusion is that so long as we get our ration of Core Sleep, consisting of Slow Wave Sleep and some REM sleep, the brain will recover from its waking wear and tear. The rest he calls 'optional sleep', which has no essential purpose but 'fills the tedious hours of darkness until sunrise, maintaining sleep beyond the point where core sleep declines', and it may in fact not be really necessary.

HOW MUCH SLEEP DO WE NEED?

The amount of sleep needed, or taken, by individual people varies enormously. There's a standard belief that eight hours is the norm, but we all know of people who need much less. Lady Thatcher is said to thrive on four or five, and there have been a number of other famous short sleepers, including Winston Churchill and Napoleon (both of whom catnapped during the day), Voltaire who only needed three hours, and Dostoyevsky, who wrote his books between 3 p.m. and 5 or 6 the next morning. I always envy short sleepers; think how much they can get done in those extra hours!

It's quite important for couples to realize that these variations are real; a short sleeper married to a long sleeper can make their partner's life quite difficult if they insist on banging around at six in the morning, or interpret the other's genuine needs as laziness.

Short and long sleepers have been found by and large to have different personalities. Short sleepers tend to be hard-working, ambitious, and rather obsessive, as well as extrovert and efficient. Long sleepers worry more, are less self-assured and value their sleep, which they may use as an escape. They are also often creative people – and creative people are said to dream more and to have more vivid and adventurous dreams than other people. Einstein was a long sleeper.

THE AGES OF SLEEP

The amount of sleep we need also varies with age. The 'average' 7.5 applies to adults between 16 and 50. Most small babies sleep about 16–18 hours a day, and toddlers still need a lot more sleep than adults. However, some older children may actually need less than adults, something which parents don't always recognize. With adolescence, the picture changes; some teenagers will sleep up to 15 hours a night. They are not necessarily being lazy, and will grow out of it. However, parents should note that longer sleeping hours are also a symptom of depression, which can hit teenagers quite badly. At about the age of 16 we reach the 'normal' adult pattern – that is, whatever is normal for us.

From the age of 40 in men and 50 in women, the pattern alters again. In some women the menopause temporarily disrupts sleeping patterns. But in everyone, as they grow older, night-time sleep becomes lighter and more broken, with fewer dreams. In addition, many older people take naps during the day, so needing less sleep at night. Including catnaps, the average sleep for 70-year-olds is about six hours in 24. It's important to realize this, since many old people ask their doctors for help with their 'insomnia' when in fact they are sleeping quite normally for their age.

YOUR BODY CLOCK: CIRCADIAN RHYTHMS

The functioning of our bodies is governed by a biological inner clock, known as the circadian rhythm (from the Latin *circa diem*, meaning 'about a day'). This regulates the times when various organs become more or less active, and when the production of various hormones peaks and tails off. The length of the circadian day is normally between 24 and 25 hours; some people have sleep problems because their body clocks are out of timing with the norm, or disturbed by things like shift work and jet lag.

The siesta, traditional in hot countries like Spain, is in decline as Mediterranean businesses come into line with the rest of Europe. Yet it could be much more natural than our own patterns. The circadian rhythm is set to bring on sleep twice a day, mainly at night, but also in the early afternoon, which is why many people feel sleepy after lunch.

The circadian rhythm also varies with age. Babies sleep regularly during the day, at first at around three-hourly intervals, tailing off to a morning and an afternoon sleep; by the age of about two and a half they are sleeping in the afternoon only. In the elderly, the need for an afternoon sleep usually returns.

It appears to be the circadian rhythm which is responsible for some people being 'owls', finding it hard to wake in the morning but lively at night, while others are 'larks', leaping out of bed first thing and drooping by ten in the evening. Interestingly, these differences seem to grow less as people age.

CHAPTER 2

Insomnia

Insomnia is defined by sleep experts as difficulty in initiating and maintaining sleep, which has continued for at least three weeks. Chronic insomnia can last for years, while intermittent insomnia can be triggered by particular anxieties or crises. People experience insomnia in different ways: for some it's the tossing and turning for what feels like hours before they drop off; others wake up at intervals and feel they never get a good night; and others wake early in the morning, and can't get off to sleep again.

Insomnia can't be measured by the number of hours you sleep, since people's needs vary so much. It's been found in sleep laboratories that some insomniacs actually sleep longer than 'normal' sleepers: if you need ten hours and only sleep for eight, then you won't feel as refreshed as the good sleeper who needs seven.

Different types of insomnia have traditionally been related to different states of mind; it's often said that not being able to get off to sleep at night is a symptom of anxiety, while waking early is a sign of depression. In fact, it's not as simple as that. Some anxious and depressed people actually sleep more, presumably in an effort to escape from their feelings. Some depressed people can't get off to sleep, and some anxious people fall asleep normally, but wake in the small hours.

A number of sleep experts believe that anger and resentment are more frequent causes of insomnia than anxiety and depression. Others suggest that the over-active, churning mind may not be a cause of insomnia, but a result. In addition, there is often more than one factor involved; an over-active mind may be related to an under-active body, for example. And as you can see from the check-list opposite, the causes are not always emotional.

Type of Problem	Possible Causes/Contributory Factors
Taking a long time to get to sleep (most common in people under 30 and women)	Habit
	Emotional stress (anxiety, depression, unhappiness, anger, guilt etc)
	Unsolved problems
	Obsessive thinking
	Psychiatric disturbances
	Dietary factors: including too many junk foods, stimulating foods and drinks, and eating heavy meals late at night.
	Digestive problems
	Smoking, especially in the evenings
	Lack of regular exercise
	Stress (at home or work)
	Major life changes – moving house, divorce, changing jobs etc.
	Certain medical conditions
	Neurological problems
	Needing less sleep than you think you do
	Napping during the day
	Jet lag, working night shifts and other body clock disturbances
	External disturbances like noise

Type of Problem	Possible Causes/Contributory Factors
Waking during the night (more common in older people and men)	As above, plus: High degrees of anger and irritability Heavy alcohol consumption Withdrawal from alcohol or drugs (medical or otherwise) Nightmares Fear of nightmares (waking just before you are about to dream) Not being fully extended during the day
Waking early and not going back to sleep	As above, plus: Severe depression Sleeping pill dependency Alcoholism
Getting 'enough' sleep but still feeling tired	Sleep apnea (a respiratory disorder) Depression Narcolepsy

QUALITY VERSUS QUANTITY

Insomnia is unpleasant. It is boring and uncomfortable in itself, and it can affect your daily activities, work and relationships. However, it may not be quite as damaging as some insomniacs fear. Sleep research laboratories have shown that people who normally sleep for seven to eight hours can adapt over time to as much as two hours' less sleep daily without impairing their mental or physical ability. And when people have been totally deprived of sleep for between eight and eleven days (the longest times so far studied) most of the body's organs, except for the brain, continue to function remarkably well. While the brain does need rest, Dr Horne stresses that 'everything else from the neck down seems to cope very well, without sleep, provided you get regular rest and regular food.'

Nevertheless, too little sleep can and does affect us, both because of genuine fatigue, but also because we *believe* that shortened sleep will cause us suffering. Our beliefs about how things should be have a major effect on how we react to them.

So, how much sleep do we really need?

Dr Horne believes that around six hours is more than adequate for mental health; any sleep after that comes into his category of 'optional sleep'. If his theory is correct, what the brain needs is Core Sleep, the deep slow-wave sleep. This should provide some reassurance to insomniacs: Core Sleep predominates during the first sleep cycles, so even if you only sleep for a few hours, you will be getting a period of this important deep sleep, together with some REM sleep.

Conditions in sleep laboratories, of course, where the human guinea-pigs are fed and rested, and have chosen to lose sleep, are quite different from those of the person tossing and turning in the lonely small hours – even if they end up getting the same amount of sleep, which is possible. EEG readings show that most insomniacs actually sleep much more than they claim to: quite often people who feel they have only slept an hour or two have actually slept for several. It appears that people's *perception* of their insomnia can cause as much stress as the insomnia itself, and it may well be that *worrying* about insomnia can make you just as stressed, tetchy and tired as not sleeping. It will also contribute to keeping you awake.

So, if you are insomniac, there are three important things to remember. Firstly, you may be getting more sleep than you think. Secondly, so long as you get some sleep and can relax your body, you will not come to long-term harm. Thirdly, your attitude towards your sleep has a lot to do with the quality of the sleep you get.

The first step towards beating insomnia is not to worry about it.

CHAPTER 3

Seeking the cause

As we've seen, there are many possible causes of insomnia not all of them emotional. It may be sensible – if you haven't already done so – to have a medical check-up with your doctor or a well-qualified complementary therapist. If you were referred to a sleep disorders clinic, you would be taken through a detailed questionnaire covering your medical history and general health, state of mind, relationships, past history, eating and drinking habits, and recent life, as well as your actual sleep patterns.

Your sleeping arrangements are also important; you'd be asked where you sleep, who with, and about your relationship with that person. (Your sleeping partner, if you have one, would probably be invited along as well.) In this way a very complete picture would be built up, in order to disentangle what's causing or contributing to your insomnia.

Sometimes quite simple answers are rapidly found – too much coffee-drinking for example. Sometimes the reasons are more worrying, like alcoholism or drug addiction. Very often the causes relate to emotional stress, including worry about the insomnia itself.

FORMULATING A STRATEGY

In a sleep clinic, once a detailed assessment has been made, a strategy would be worked out with you for improving your sleep. If you were found to be severely depressed, drug therapy might be recommended for a time. And of course if you were found to be suffering from a medical, neurological or psychiatric illness, you would be referred for appropriate treatment.

For most people, the options could include relaxation training, or a behavioural programme to restructure your sleeping habits. Or you might be referred to a psychiatrist or a clinical psychologist to help you deal with emotional stress. Psychological help might take the practical form of helping you to deal with anxiety by sorting out your priorities. You might be considered a suitable candidate for cognitive therapy, a way of learning how to change negative and anxious thoughts and beliefs about yourself. You might be helped by hypnotherapy, which a few psychiatrists and psychologists practise; or it might be considered that you would benefit from psychotherapy. We'll be looking at some of these options in the next few chapters.

SLEEPING PILLS (A LAST RESORT)

Publicity about the side-effects of sleeping pills and tranquilizers belonging to the benzodiazepine group of drugs has made the general public wary of taking them, and doctors wary of prescribing them. When they were first produced in the 1960s they seemed to answer all sorts of problems: now we know that these drugs don't solve any problems, and can be extremely addictive.

In addition, when taken as sleeping pills, benzodiazepines reduce the quality of your sleep. They cause suppression of REM sleep in the first part of the night, often with a rebound effect with more dreaming later in the night, which can cause early wakening. They can also leave people feeling fuzzy-minded next morning, which is particularly dangerous in the old, since it can make them confused and increases the risk of falls. Unfortunately, no really satisfactory alternative sleeping pill has yet been produced.

There may be a case for taking medication for a day or two under certain conditions – after the shock of a bereavement, for instance. But no one should take sleeping pills for year after year, as has been the case in the past.

Practitioners of natural therapies can be very supportive in helping you to come off sleeping pills (which should always be done gradually), or dealing with the after-effects of coming off. They are not allowed to recommend you to go against your doctor's advice; you can of course make your own decision, but it's best if you work in co-operation with your GP. Some natural practitioners prefer people to give up before starting treatment with them, either because the drugs may interfere with their treatment, or because they like to know that the patient is committed to stopping.

What natural practitioners can supply is the time and the listening ear that busy GPs are rarely able to give, together with natural treatments to strengthen and detoxify the body. A naturopath and osteopath tells me that about 5 per cent of her patients are hooked on sleeping pills when they come to her. They usually come for treatment for some other problem, and after a while ask for her help in giving up the pills. She has found it possible to help them by using herbal pills as a bridge, and combining counselling with her physical treatments.

On giving up benzodiazepines, some people experience increased fatigue for a time, and some increased agitation. There can also be a period of increased dreaming. And it can happen that the suppressed anxieties for which they originally took the pills start surfacing. This is easier to cope with if you accept it as part of the healing process rather than a sign of sickness: it shows that these feelings are now on their way out. Counselling from a professional counsellor or alternative practitioner can help you through this stage.

HERBAL SEDATIVES

Practitioners of natural therapies would much rather help you to solve your sleeping problems altogether than be dependent on medication, but herbal tranquillizers can be useful and safe as a temporary prop while you recover your normal sleep.

Over 90 sedative herbal pills can currently be bought over the counter at health food shops and some chemists. Most of them contain slightly differing proportions of the same ingredients including valerian, scullcap, passiflora, wild lettuce and other sleep-inducing herbs. They can be taken during the day to counteract anxiety as well as to help you sleep at night.

Most herbal remedies are very mild, without the mind-deadening effect that chemical tranquillizers can induce, and they are not technically addictive; however it is possible to become psychologically dependent on them. While preferable to chemical drugs, there is still a risk of using them as a substitute for really dealing with your insomnia, and taken regularly for a few weeks on the trot their effectiveness can be reduced.

Herbal pills in general have no side-effects, and are safe to take; their sale is supervised by the Committee of Safety on Medicines. However, very occasionally, a person has an individual allergic reaction to a herbal product, which does not mean that it is dangerous to the rest of the population. In choosing pills, your health food store manager should be able to give you some guidance.

For further information about herbal remedies, see the sections on Bedtime Drinks in Chapter 12, and on Medical Herbalism in Chapter 13.

CHAPTER 4

The habit of insomnia

Whatever the cause or causes of your insomnia, sleeplessness is nearly always a symptom of some kind of disharmony in your daytime life. This disharmony may be mental, emotional, physical or environmental, often a combination. But whatever it is, it needs to be faced and dealt with during the day. By the time you get to bed, it's really too late.

Poor sleep can be exacerbated by bad eating and drinking habits, lack of exercise, and other physical and environmental factors which contribute further to tension and stress. We'll be looking at all of these in due course. But since your physical habits usually reflect your view of yourself, let's look first at the mental and emotional side.

The most important thing is to realize that you *can* do something. To decide what to do, you will need to look at your attitudes and lifestyle and possibly ask yourself a few questions. But once you start on a plan of action you will not only improve your sleep pattern but start creating for yourself a happier, more satisfying daytime life. As you read on, note what applies to you, and what you personally can change.

SLEEP AND HABIT

If your insomnia has become severe enough or prolonged enough for you to be reading this book, then it is in part a habit, perhaps alongside some other habits, like not looking after yourself well enough, or postponing dealing with anxieties. And short-term insomnia can become long-term insomnia simply by acquiring the habit of expecting to sleep badly.

Human beings are odd creatures: most of us like to think we are independent, free-thinking spirits. Yet a surprising amount of our behaviour is totally conditioned, starting when we are very young. Much of our conditioning is helpful and life-supporting; it would be very inconvenient if every time you crossed a road you had to relearn the desirability of looking both ways, or what red, amber and green lights mean. Unfortunately the mechanical part of our brain absorbs other, less helpful lessons, like associating bed with lying awake.

It's common these days for the brain to be likened to a computer – a computer more vast and complex than any yet built, and of course with a capacity for original thought, but nonetheless a machine which obediently reproduces whatever programming is fed into it.

Thus a few people are 'sleep hypochondriacs'; early in life an over-anxious parent has programmed them with the idea that without eight hours' solid sleep their health will suffer. The computer part of the brain that has accepted this belief reacts with anxiety when those solid eight hours aren't forthcoming – until the owner of the computer takes a fresh look at the old programme and decides to delete it and feed in new, up-to-date information.

SELF TALK

The best way to break unhelpful habits is to start exchanging them for helpful ones. The first thing is to recognize in what particular ways your habitual thinking or behaviour is keeping you in that sleepless groove. How do you talk to yourself and others about sleep? If you label yourself 'insomniac' and tell yourself every time you head for bed that it'll take you ages to get to sleep, you are simply reinforcing the programming that keeps you awake. You can change some of that thinking now, by telling yourself that you are now on the way to improving your sleep, and by no longer telling other people that you suffer from insomnia.

Be honest with yourself about this. Lots of people 'enjoy' their ailments. In some cases this can be an excuse for avoiding things they don't want to do, or even living a more fulfilled life. I would stress that this kind of pattern is very rarely deliberate: it's often another conditioned response, perhaps going back to a time when being ill got a child more of its mother's love and attention than when he or she was well. Never sleeping well may prevent people like this from facing up to other problems, or taking on new ventures which would mean change. That doesn't mean they are purposefully choosing not to sleep, but it's possible that lack of sleep has secondary advantages, like making their families feel sorry for them.

Could this apply to you? And if it does, do you really want to be someone others feel sorry for? Close your eyes and imagine for a moment telling your spouse or workmates, 'I slept wonderfully last night!' How does it feel? Probably uncomfortable at this moment, because it isn't true. How comfortable would it feel if it were true?

Start noticing your habitual thoughts about insomnia. In particular, look out for sentences beginning 'I always …' or 'I never …' or 'I know …' For example:

'I always take hours to get to sleep' or *'I always wake up for hours in the middle of the night'*.

These statements may not actually be true, although they feel true to you. As we've seen, most insomniacs over-estimate how long they take to get to sleep or lie awake during the night. You could make a start by recognizing that your perception of the amount of sleep you get may be inaccurate.

'*I'm never going to get to sleep tonight*' is another habitual statement which is an excellent way of programming your brain to stay awake.

'*I know I'll feel dreadful if I can't get to sleep.*' Of course, lack of sleep makes you tired, but you can also talk yourself into feeling worse. There are alternatives, such as telling yourself that even though you'd like more sleep, your body is still getting all the rest it needs.

Make a game of catching these kinds of thoughts. It may help you to write them down. Then try replacing your negative statements with positive ones; a good start might be: 'I'm now learning how to sleep better.' Make your positive statements ones you can believe. Telling yourself 'I am going to sleep perfectly tonight' may not work, because at this point you probably won't believe it, and trying to convince yourself will set up further tension.

But you could try: 'I will take tonight as it comes.' You may be surprised by the results.

Starting to change your self-talk can be a way of opening up other possibilities. Once you realize that you don't have to be a victim of your own thinking and reactions, all kinds of barriers can begin to crumble.

CHANGING THE PATTERN

A popular way of treating insomnia today is a behavioural psychology method called stimulus-control, which consists of retraining yourself to sleep by learning to associate bed and bedtime with sleep, and sleep alone. This is the routine:

1. Use your bed and bedroom for sleep only. Don't watch television, listen to the radio, read, work, smoke or eat in bed. Making love is of course permitted!

2. Always get up at the same time, including weekends and holidays. Lie-ins may be tempting, but if you take more sleep than you need on Sunday morning it'll be harder to get to sleep on Sunday night.

   If you find waking up really difficult, place your alarm clock at the other side of the room so that you have to get up to turn it off. Put the light on straight away, as light can stimulate wakefulness.

3. Don't take naps during the day. You can overcome post-lunch sleepiness with some deep breathing, or a quick walk round the block.

4. Don't go to bed until you are really sleepy.

5. If you don't fall asleep within ten minutes, get up and do something else *in another room*. Don't go back to bed until you are ready to fall asleep.

There are further sleep-assisting habits you can develop:

1. Deal with specific anxieties during the day or early evening.

2. Avoid stimulating foods and drinks in the evening. These include coffee, tea and alcohol. Smoking is also a stimulant; if you can't give it up immediately, at least cut down, especially in the evening.

3. Avoid stimulating activities late at night, including strenuous exercise, work and arguments.

4. Establish a winding-down routine before you go to bed. Spend the last hour before bedtime preparing for sleep, including some relaxation and a warm bath. (There's more about winding-down in Chapter 12.)

5. Make sure your bedroom is both well-aired and warm.

A WORD ABOUT NAPS

For good sleepers, daytime naps can be beneficial and restorative; as we've seen, the human body clock actually seems built for sleep twice a day. However, while you are recovering a normal sleep pattern, naps are best avoided. The exception here would be parents of new babies, who are not technically insomniac, but are getting broken nights. If you are elderly and the need for a daytime nap becomes overpowering, take it but remember to allow for less sleep at night.

CHAPTER 5

Restoring the balance

Our brains aren't purely computers. The human brain is divided in two, like a walnut, and each half has specific functions. As a rule the left hemisphere controls the right side of the body, and deals with functions like speech and logical thinking. The right hemisphere, controlling the left side of the body, is responsible for abstract thought, dreaming, intuition, and visual imagery. In a few people, the sides are reversed.

To be in harmony with ourselves, both sides of the brain need to be equally active, and to work in co-operation with each other. In this hectic world most people use the logical side most of the time, at the expense of the intuitive, imaginative side. To restore the balance, the day-dreaming part of our minds needs to be exercised as much as the logical part.

A left–right imbalance is often reflected in the physical

body; people can be quite lop-sided without realizing it, because they are putting all their energies into one aspect of themselves. Alternative therapies like osteopathy, kinesiology and the Alexander Technique can help to correct this.

The intuitive hemisphere has been called the gateway to the unconscious; through it we can get in touch with our creativity and inspiration, our hidden desires, needs, memories, and inner wisdom. It is this side of the brain that comes up with brilliant flashes of intuition, or solutions to problems that logic has been unable to solve. Have you ever found that when you stop worrying about a problem and let it go, the answer just pops in – sometimes during a dream, sometimes when you wake up in the morning? Quietening the chatter of the logical brain gives the creative side a chance to help us.

Yet we have been taught to neglect it. You could compare the two hemispheres to a hard-working, serious-minded parent, and a creative child who wants to play. The parent concentrates on telling the child how to behave, and doesn't listen to what it has to say. Yet given a chance, the creative child can come up with original ideas and solutions that the conformist parent hasn't considered.

When mind and body are allowed to relax, the activity of the two hemispheres starts to equalize. At the same time, the brain-waves slow down from the active, busy beta rate, producing the alpha-rhythm that normally precedes sleep. We become both more peaceful and more creative.

This state of mind can be achieved in a number of ways, for instance through relaxation and meditation (which I'll be returning to in Chapter 10), and through the use of mental imagery, including hypnotherapy, self-hypnosis and visualization.

HYPNOTHERAPY

Hypnotherapy is not a simple process of telling you that you will sleep well, or stop smoking, or eat less. A good hypnotherapist will need to know why you are not sleeping, and will help you to tackle the problems underlying your insomnia, before going on to help you make inner changes to achieve more control over your own behaviour.

Under hypnosis you reach that relaxed, dreamy (but not usually unconscious) state in which suggestions can be more readily received by your right brain, bypassing the disbelieving left brain. It has sometimes had remarkable results in healing the physical body, and can be very helpful in the relief of pain. But your mind will only receive those suggestions it is willing to receive.

Hypnotherapists work in a variety of ways, but will normally start by taking your case history and discussing your current problems. They have their own favourite methods of helping you to relax, perhaps by counting down slowly from ten to one, or by asking you to take yourself in imagination to a peaceful, pleasant place – perhaps a country scene, or the seaside, imagining the sights, colours, scents and sounds.

In this relaxed state, with the logical brain on hold, the therapist can help you review your anxieties and fears in a safe atmosphere. He or she may help you to discover those other, more helpful parts of yourself that have been repressed, and explore ways of making changes in your life. This can be quite an enjoyable game, in which you imagine new scenarios with yourself as both actor and director.

Hypnotherapy can be very useful if you suffer from recurrent bad dreams or nightmares. A hypnotherapist can help you to discover what those dreams are trying to tell you, and resolve the tension that keeps them recurring. It is also possible to learn to take an active part in one's dreams and so gain some control over them. Challenging and overcoming a fearful figure or event in a dream can have a big spin-off effect on your self-esteem and ability to control your own destiny.

SELF-HYPNOSIS AND VISUALIZATION

The imagination can have a direct effect on the body, for good or ill. When you imagine or remember a disaster, your pulse can start racing and your breathing can become more shallow, as the body's stress system starts revving up. It doesn't matter that the disaster isn't real: your body and nervous system react as though it is. Similarly, when you imagine yourself healthy and happy, your body starts to feel healthier and stronger.

In a relaxed, day-dreaming state, you can mentally picture the outcome that you want, whether it's better sleep, or confidently taking and passing your driving test. It's important to believe and expect that what you visualize will come about. In so doing, you are using an in-depth way of reprogramming your mental computer.

Visualization techniques may not be right for everyone: if you are an anxious striver, you may put too much effort into what should be effortless, or make yourself worse by focusing on symptoms rather than health. But even if you don't use specific techniques, you are using the power of thought and imagination throughout the day, both mentally and verbally. All the more reason to exchange depressing thoughts about your life and your sleep for positive ideas about what you really want.

For successful self-hypnosis, the first, essential step is to be able to relax deeply. If you are normally tense, you may need some help in learning to relax sufficiently. (See Chapter 10 for more about relaxation.) Some people have successfully taught themselves to visualize from books; there are also some good tapes on the market which can start you off, though it's not a good idea to rely on them for the rest of your life. For most people it's easier initially to be taught by someone else.

THOUGHT AND ENERGY

Human beings are more than their physical bodies. We also consist of a complete energy system: the energy-field surrounding the body (often referred to as the aura), together with channels of energy flowing through the body and a number of major energy centres (also called chakras) which relate to the endocrine glands.

Although invisible to most people, the energy system can be seen by some psychics and healers, and physically sensed by many healers and natural therapists. Many of those who work directly on the body, like manipulative therapists, massage practitioners and healers, can help to rebalance your energies, and will encourage you to maintain that balance.

The healer Betty Shine stresses the importance of the energy of the mind, which she sees as separate from that around the body. In her book *Mind to Mind* (Corgi, 1989) she describes how, when someone is depressed, the mind energy funnels down like a black cloud, compressing the physical organs and eventually impeding their healthy functioning; conversely, when someone thinks happy, positive thoughts, she can see the mind energy radiating outwards like a halo, lifting depression from the physical system.

Most healers and health practitioners agree that your thoughts have a direct effect on your body and energy system, which is worth bearing in mind next time you start brooding about something unpleasant. In fact, many go further: thoughts, they say, are forms of energy which, if focused on often enough, will take material form. This helps to explain why people who expect disasters very often get them, and why it's important to exchange negative views of life for positive ones.

CHAPTER 6

The churning mind

Probably the most common complaint among poor sleepers is difficulty in getting off to sleep. It's almost always related to a mind that won't switch itself off. Your thoughts go round and round, you toss and turn, and an hour later you're tired, twitchy, and wide awake.

The churning mind may be caused by anxiety about something specific – an exam, a job interview, a work project, a partner's illness, or the state of your finances. It is possibly caused even more often by resentment or anger, brooding over unpleasant events, sometimes from the recent past, sometimes from way back. You relive the scenes, inventing scenarios in which you find just the right words to put down that person who insulted you yesterday, or even years ago. Or you may be feeling depressed and lonely, wishing your life were different, blaming yourself or others because it isn't, and replaying past regrets, missed opportunities, or lost happiness.

A great deal of night-time churning is connected with unfinished business, something that computer in your head can't stand. It chugs away looking for solutions, and won't shut up. Or it allows you to get to sleep, and then wakes you up with a bad dream to remind you of a problem, or to tell you, 'Hey, we really must do some worrying about this!'

Regularly waking with nightmares or bad dreams can make you anxious about going to bed in the first place; usually these, too, concern unfinished business. Night terrors – suddenly waking from non-dreaming sleep with a sense of fear and doom – are often the result of past traumas. Recurring dreams, too, may stem from traumatic past events – car crashes, a battering spouse, or an assault – which the conscious mind has tried to forget. But the unconscious mind is still trying to cope with it in the only way it knows how. In such cases it is important to seek professional help from a counsellor, psychotherapist or hypnotherapist who can help you to heal your fears, so that they no longer fester and cause you misery.

Some people aren't particularly worried about anything, but just have very active minds. Many of them accept this, often creative people who come up with creative ideas as they lie awake. But if your thoughts are unpleasant, sad or anxious, they are crying out to be dealt with.

Bed is not the place to deal with them.

WHO'S IN THE DRIVING SEAT?

Rushing round all day and going to bed with a mind that's exhausted but awake is all too common these days. Modern life doesn't encourage natural rhythms. We start work at the same time all year round, whether it's dark or light; commuter travel is uncomfortable and frustrating. Office atmospheres are often unhealthy as well as fraught; lunch may be a snatched sandwich or hamburger. For many people 'relaxation' takes place in the artificial atmosphere and noise of pubs and discos.

Small wonder that rushers-round can't sleep. The whole physical and nervous system becomes jangled and out of gear. There is no breathing space to look at problems – or just to breathe! Body and mind are poorly nourished. And underlying this frantic rush, an anxious little voice is often sending anxious little messages that we don't want to hear – 'Am I good enough?' – 'Is this all there is to life?' – 'Why aren't I happy?'

If your life is anything like this, and it has resulted in insomnia, ask yourself what you are truly getting out of it. OK, so modern life is like that. But does that mean *yours* has to be? What or who is driving you to over-work, eat badly, maybe drink too much, or work till all hours so that by bedtime your brain is buzzing?

Much of our busy-busy behaviour is due to conditioning by other people, and our beliefs about how life should be lived may be nothing to do with what we really need. The work ethic says we mustn't waste a moment; social standards say we must have a 'good time' and be successful. We must also be *seen* to be successful by buying and owning more and more goodies for ourselves and our families; to keep the merry-go-round turning we have to work even harder. Yet when you were a child, was this what you wanted from life? Who programmed your computer?

Our beliefs come from a number of different sources, which is why they often conflict. Some psychotherapists point out that we all have multiple personalities, often referred to as sub-personalities or 'voices'. For example, most people have an inner critic sitting in judgement on their every action; at the same time there's an inner child, made to feel small by the critic's remarks. Many of us have an inner saboteur, doing its best to make us make a mess of things. But there are other parts of us which often don't get a look in – for example, a wise self, a peaceful self, and a creative child who wants to play.

So, try listening to the thoughts and voices underlying your daily rush. Who's driving you on? Are you

responding to other people's programming – perhaps
a critical father demanding that you prove your worth,
or a perfectionist mother setting you impossibly high
standards? Do you have to believe those voices from the
past? What does the real you need and want from life, and
are you getting it?

DEALING WITH SPECIFIC PROBLEMS

If you're being kept awake by specific problems, learn
to deal with them during the day, so that you don't take
unfinished business to bed with you.

Find some time during the day or early evening to write
a list of the worries or anxieties that are keeping you
awake. A friend of mine who did this realized she had
one 'super-anxiety', around which revolved a set of sub-
anxieties. Once she'd taken steps to deal with the super-
anxiety, many of the sub-anxieties were automatically
cleared up, and the rest became much less important.

Having identified the super-anxiety, write down what you can do about it. If you're worried about a job interview, what steps can you take to prepare yourself for it? If getting a job interview is difficult, what can you do about it? Are there any alternatives to the kind of action you've been taking so far?

Once you've decided on your course of action, close your eyes for a few minutes and see yourself taking it. If you are anxious about a forthcoming event, or finally doing that thing you've been nervous about, picture yourself dealing with it calmly and efficiently; don't imagine all the difficulties in the way, but see the successful end-product. Set the scene very clearly: see yourself with your problem solved or having achieved the thing you fear doing. Imagine telling someone about it, and hearing their congratulations. Don't worry if you can't visualize clearly; imagine how you'll feel – relieved, pleased with yourself, no longer anxious. In this way you are priming your brain with the fact that solutions are possible; anxiety or hesitation are not the only options.

Then close your notebook, and put it in a drawer for the night, knowing *you have done everything you can.* Physically putting your list away tells the anxious or worried part of your mind that that's it for today, thank you! You are also making space for the more creative part of your mind to come up with solutions, possibly during sleep.

Then, having identified what action to take, *do it*! It's amazing how anxiety and fear disappear and depression lifts when you actually get going on a project. The mind can't focus on two things at once. Actors who suffer from stagefright lose it when they walk on the stage and begin concentrating on their roles. If you are really involved in and concentrated on an activity, there isn't room for negative feelings.

Supposing, for some reason, there is no direct action you can take to deal with the problem itself? *What you can do right now* is to take physical action to deal with your state of anxiety, depression or lethargy.

LOOKING AFTER YOUR BODY

Anxiety, depression, and obsessive thinking all have a strong physical component, since they trigger the production of stress hormones which create further anxiety, depression and obsessive thinking. Breaking the cycle by looking after your body will have a positive feedback on your emotions.

Stress hormones are actually produced to gear us up for action. If you start taking regular exercise you will get rid of them healthily. You have to make a commitment, says my 'super-anxiety' friend; part of her strategy was to go swimming every day. She had to force herself to go to the pool for the first few days, but it was worth it; feeling physically relaxed and well helped her to get back in control.

CHAPTER 7

Your sleep and other people

Some sleep experts believe that anger and resentment are more common causes of night-time churning than anxiety or depression. If that's the case with you, it's important to drop them, for the sake of your sleep. It is possible!

If you're angry about a current situation, either accept it or do something about it; otherwise all that negative energy (and there's a lot of energy in anger) will go on keeping you awake.

Many people fear confrontations, but it is possible to say what you feel about a situation without having a violent explosion. Telling the person or people concerned calmly how you feel about their behaviour, without blaming or accusing them, can often open up better communications.

If you can't confront the person, or if the anger-making situation is in the past, whether it's last week or several years ago, tell yourself that whatever anybody else has said or done, however unfair, cruel, snide, or dishonest, it's over now. While you are brooding, going over the scene or scenes, rehearsing the remarks you could have made, or intend to make in the future, the other person may well have forgotten the whole thing. The only person who's making you angry now is you, every time you mentally relive those scenes.

In addition, if you accept the suggestion that thought is energy, consider this: what we think comes back to us. It is generally accepted in healing and spiritual groups that when we send thoughts of healing and kindness to other people, not only will those people benefit but so will we. Thoughts of resentment and vengeance may not affect other people at all, unless it's to make them even more unpleasant; but they most certainly will boomerang back at us.

There are other considerations in storing anger. You are not only keeping yourself awake. Firstly, you are setting yourself up for physical problems: high blood pressure, heart problems and arthritis are among the side-effects of long-harboured anger. Secondly, when you let someone else's behaviour rule your thoughts, emotions and sleep, you are making the person responsible for your peace of mind, handing over to them your personal autonomy.

Resentment is often a deeply ingrained habit, but it's one we may have been taught by others. Small children are naturally forgiving; I suspect that some of us learn to be resentful from our elders. It's an unhealthy habit, and once you've given it up you will feel better all round.

Anger creates the tense muscles that give you headaches and shoulder pain, as well as stimulating the release of stress hormones, all of which can contribute to your insomnia. Do try to get it physically out of your system, during the day.

One way is the famous pillow-bashing technique, which really does work. Find a time and a place where you can be alone, and make a pillow the focus of your anger. Don't think of it as the person you are angry with: you are not trying to hurt anyone else but to heal yourself.

Start thumping. Yell at the same time. Really let go, and keep shouting and thumping until you are exhausted, drained of your angry feelings, and with your shoulders and arms released of all that tension.

The next stage is to forgive the person or people in question. That can be a hard one, but the important thing is your willingness to forgive. Forgiveness doesn't mean that you condone bad behaviour, or that you have to let anyone continue to treat you badly; it means that you are wiping your own slate clean and getting the past out of your system.

Visualization techniques can be helpful here. In a relaxed state you can visualize the other person, possibly attached to you by cords that your thoughts and feelings have created. See yourself cutting through those cords and then burning them, freeing you both. Or imagine a conversation in which you tell the person that you're releasing them from your thoughts. It may help to imagine them apologizing to you.

Another approach is to imagine your mind as a

beautiful room, in which you have the right to entertain the guests of your choice. At the moment it's full of these cross, grumbling people, reminding you you've been hard done by. Tell them you don't enjoy their company, and show them the door. If they're reluctant to leave, sweep them out with a broom. Your room is now empty and clean, and there is space in it for more welcome visitors, including peace of mind, serenity and better sleep. Show them in and make them at home.

A lot of depressed people suffer from guilt and anger towards themselves, quite often for no good reason. If you belong to this group, do be kind to yourself. Forgive yourself as you would forgive anyone else. Use visualization to let go of those feelings and start afresh, reminding yourself of all the good things about you.

PARTNERSHIP PROBLEMS

Most marriages and partnerships go through bad patches; feeling resentful towards your partner can be a major source of sleeplessness. Do try to resolve your problems, or at least start to, during the day or early evening; don't leave it until bedtime to have rows. And don't lie in bed brooding over your partner's faults and telling yourself that if only he or she were different you would be quite happy.

You cannot change other people; what you can do is to tell them how you feel – they may have no idea. And give them the opportunity to tell you how they feel. People often make totally false assumptions about what's going on in someone else's head, even their nearest and dearest. Talking openly and honestly, and listening to the other person's point of view as well as expressing your own, can clear the air remarkably at times.

Women often have difficulty in acknowledging that they are angry at all; we are still brought up with the idea that anger isn't very nice. Some women repress their own wants and needs in order to be perfect wives and mothers; they don't realize that underneath they are quite angry at constantly giving out to others. This kind of situation can trigger insomnia. If you are constantly giving out, make sure that you get your own needs met as well.

It has been found helpful for couples to have a regular weekly date and time for expressing their grievances in turn, and listening to each other without interruption while they express them. End the session by telling your partner what you appreciate about them; couples often neglect this. You hear people say, 'I don't have to tell my wife/husband I love her/him, she/he knows without me telling her/him.' I think that's an awful pity. It doesn't matter whether we know or not, it's always heart-warming to be told.

When you live with someone else it can be a good idea to have a spare bed ready made up, or a sofa, to which one of you can retire when you both need space. (Don't retire to it forever, though, if you want to keep the relationship going.)

In some of the books and articles I've read about insomnia, the writers remark gaily that sex is the one activity it's good to indulge in before bedtime, the assumption being that you then drop off, happy and relaxed.

What if you don't? An unsatisfactory sexual relationship can leave at least one partner feeling worse off than with no sex at all. As with all the other problems causing insomnia, it's important to do something about it. The longer difficulties build up the more insoluble they can seem.

If you have a good relationship and goodwill on both sides, and if your partner agrees, ask your doctor to put you in touch with a sex therapist (unfortunately they're not easily available on the NHS), or get in touch with a marriage guidance counsellor. If there's no real goodwill, of course, you need to ask yourself why you are staying in this marriage. Again, it can be helpful to see a marriage guidance or some other kind of counsellor, to help you to clarify the confused feelings that are keeping you awake.

CHAPTER 8

A healthy environment

Ideally, your bedroom should be associated with sleep, and not with other activities. It should also be warm and welcoming, with a peaceful and healthy atmosphere; some bedrooms, as will be seen, can actually damage your health.

COLOURS

Colours have an influence not only on our visual sense but on our nervous system; they radiate at different wavelengths, some of which are stimulating, and some calming. Calming colours for bedrooms are soft blues and greens, pastel pinks and peaches; neutral colours like beige and cream are also appropriate. Avoid vivid colours, particularly in a child's bedroom, where they might seem cheerful but can be over-stimulating.

THE BED

Your bed should obviously be comfortable, ideally with
a firm but not over-hard mattress. People's tastes in
mattresses vary, and if you're happy with a squashy one,
that's fine. But soft mattresses are not good for your back
in the long run.

It's best to sleep with a single pillow, which keeps your
neck at a natural angle. A stiff neck is often greatly
improved when two or three pillows are replaced with a
single one. (It's been suggested, incidentally, that if you
sleep badly in strange houses, taking a familiar pillow with
you will provide the link with home that will allow sleep
to come.) Some people find hop- or herb-filled pillows
help them to sleep; you can get them at herbalists like
Culpeper's. Make sure you like the smell before buying.

FRESH, CLEAN AIR

Fresh air is important, provided it doesn't make the room
too cold. If you don't like sleeping with an open window,
consider getting an ioniser. Ionisers replace in the

atmosphere negative ions, electrically charged molecules
which are found in abundance in mountain air and around
waterfalls, and which keep the air healthy and clean.

CRYSTALS

Crystals are getting very popular these days as aids to
healing, meditation, and clearing the atmosphere. If the idea
appeals to you, rose quartz and amethyst are both considered
suitable stones for sleep; keep one by your bedside. When
you buy a crystal, it should be thoroughly cleansed before
you use it, since crystals absorb energies from the
atmosphere around them. Soak it for several hours in a
bowl of salt water, rinse it under the cold tap, don't wipe
it with a cloth but place it to dry on a sunny window sill.

IS YOUR BEDROOM HEALTHY?

Over the last few years complaints of headaches, skin
rashes, nausea, lethargy, depression, stress and fatigue have

been related to 'sick building syndrome'. The health of workers in modern buildings has been affected by factors like artificial lighting, static electricity from synthetic furniture and fabrics, low frequency electromagnetic radiation from electronic machinery, and airborne particles. Air-conditioning and non-openable windows further deplete the atmosphere of negative ions.

We don't hear too much about 'sick bedrooms', but some of these factors can also affect your home, particularly if you are sensitive. Though it's unlikely that your bedroom will be full of computers, an increasing number of synthetic fabrics are used in furnishings, bedlinen and nightwear, while harmful gas can be given off by insulation materials, lacquers, glues and vinyls. There is also increasing evidence that radiation from electric pylons can affect the health of people living near them.

So, use natural fabrics in your bedroom furnishings, linen and nightwear; and don't have a TV set in there. Although single items of electrical and electronic equipment are said to give off safe levels of radiation, we are increasingly exposed to radiation of all kinds, and the accumulation from various sources can ultimately get to us. It's also best not to use an electric blanket; if you do, switch it off and unplug it before going to bed.

CHAPTER 9

Balancing your lifestyle

If you've read this far, you will probably have identified
the causes of your insomnia, and some possible solutions.
It's often said that it takes three weeks to change a habit.
How long it will take you to break your habit of not
sleeping I can't say – it may be sooner than you think. But
three weeks is a good length of time to get yourself into a
new rhythm of life and adopt habits which will help you
towards acquiring a new, healthy sleep pattern.

Firstly, here's a check-list of some of the ground covered
so far:

- Get a physical check-up if it seems appropriate.
- Stop thinking of yourself as insomniac, and start
  seeing yourself as well on the way to good sleep.

- Get up at the same time every day; don't nap during the day, or take lie-ins. Go to bed only when you feel sleepy.

- Notice how you talk to yourself, and start rebuilding your beliefs about both your sleep and yourself.

- Practise letting go of feelings that keep you awake, like anger and resentment, helping yourself with mental imagery.

- If you have unresolved problems, make a commitment during the next three weeks to finish unfinished business by taking action *during the day*, including getting help if you need it.

In this part of the book we'll be looking at ways of making your daytime life more conducive to night time sleep, including:

- Creating more fulfilment in your life.

- Getting regular non-competitive exercise appropriate to your needs and age.

- Learning to relax or meditate, and to include some relaxation time in your daytime as well as night-time routine.

- Making sure you have a healthy diet geared to sleeping well.

- Winding down in the evenings and preparing yourself for peaceful sleep.

BEING KIND TO YOURSELF

Perhaps most importantly of all, now's the time to start treating yourself kindly. We're often told how important it is to love ourselves; many insomniacs, it seems, suffer from low self-esteem. If you've never felt really loved or valued, 'loving yourself' can seem like a tall order – or perhaps like a pat solution without much real meaning.

What it involves is simply respecting and valuing yourself as highly as you would any other human being, and behaving accordingly.

Loving yourself is yet another habit that can be cultivated. It may take time, and you may need help, perhaps by joining a therapy or assertiveness group. Meanwhile, simply start by treating yourself as kindly as you would like others to treat you.

If you have negative feelings towards yourself, they may well have been implanted there when you were a child. Imagine that you are now given the care of that child: talk to it lovingly, and appreciate all the good things about it. When you hear the voice of that inner critic in your head, tell it firmly that that is an old programme you no longer need.

GETTING INTO THE DRIVING SEAT

Whatever the cause of your insomnia, if you want to sleep better at night, it's time to get into the driving seat and decide where you really want to go. What's missing from your life that would give you some real joy or peace of mind? Whatever it is needs to provide a contrast with your daily routine, not *more* of the same.

If you're a rusher-round, make time to do something totally unconnected with work. Do you do anything creative? Could you spend more time with your family – or less, if you're constantly fulfilling their needs? Are you really doing what you want to do, or have you some unfulfilled dream that your busy lifestyle, or those inner voices, have so far prevented you from achieving? If so, what first step can you take towards it?

If you're the unadventurous type, what could you do over this three-week period that would be a real challenge? Write a list of possibilities, things you've maybe thought of doing – if you only had the confidence. (They could include signing on at a self-assertion class.)

I'm not suggesting that you instantly chuck your job and family and go off to paint in Tahiti, like Gauguin. But we sometimes deny ourselves what we really want by telling ourselves it's impossible. Or we find perfectly reasonable excuses for not getting it, either because the idea of change is threatening, or we've simply got into the habit of self-denial.

Include in your list everything you haven't done but would like to do. Be as fantastic as you like -- if a journey to the moon comes to mind, write it down. At this stage, simply allow the ideas to flow, and if a critical inner voice jumps in to tell you not to be so silly, thank it and tell it it's your life, and you're in charge.

When you've written everything you can think of, look at that list as if it had been written by another person whom you are helping. What is really possible? Maybe it's too late to become a prima donna or ballerina: but perhaps you could join a singing or dancing class (either of which would help you to sleep by using your energy in a healthy way). You want to write a novel, but feel you're not talented enough? You'll never know until you've written it. You'd like a more exciting social life, but you never get any invitations? Remember, you're in the driving seat: take the first step and ask round the people you'd like to see more of.

Rushers-round may need less activity in their schedule, not more. You may be so strongly conditioned towards constant *doing* that 'doing nothing' doesn't appear on your list; it may actually be quite scary. Yet 'doing nothing', allowing yourself a little space, to think, to day-dream, to enjoy a walk in nature, may be just what's missing.

If you are depressed, it is really important to start moving, whether your depression is due to those inner voices, or to outer circumstances. If it's caused by unhappy life events like bereavement, redundancy, or divorce, it's a natural response. You need to go through the grieving process before you feel fully yourself again; this can be true after a relationship breaks up just as much as following a death. But don't allow it to go on forever. Some people seem to stay stuck in their grief. If this is your case, it's important to take action to move yourself out of the slough of despond: to leave the unhappy past behind and take on new ventures – a new job, or voluntary work, a new hobby, or any interest that will move you forward and open up new horizons.

Perhaps your depression is due to life circumstances, such as unemployment, or the loneliness of being a single mother with small children. Don't let depression hold you back from helping yourself. Write down the aspects of your life that are making you unhappy. What can be changed? Can you get together with other people in the same boat to support each other, or join a self-help group? Make some kind of move, however small.

Perhaps you are depressed simply because you're depressed: you don't like or love yourself much. Make a point of *behaving* as if you do. Depressed people often skip meals and don't bother about looking after their surroundings. A good start to defeating your negative inner voices is to look after yourself: include in your new programme a commitment to preparing proper meals and eating them slowly. Invite yourself to a particularly nice meal once a week; give yourself treats. Keep your bedroom and bedlinen tidy, fresh and clean, as if for a valued guest.

As I've said earlier, sometimes it's necessary to get help. It is not a sign of weakness to see a counsellor or psychotherapist. You've only got to listen to the radio phone-ins to agony aunts and uncles to realize that you're not alone in needing help – and also, how helpful even a few minutes with a professional can be. Maybe getting help could be included on your list.

PLAYTIME

Most of our activities have a secondary purpose: to earn a living or keep the family and household going. One of the greatest pleasures of creative activities is doing them simply for their own sake, because you enjoy them.

An awful lot of our spare-time entertainment consists of watching other people in action, on television, at the cinema or sports matches. How much time do you spend actually *doing* something really enjoyable? Most people have a creative side which doesn't always get a look in.

Whether you're over-stressed or not stressed enough, there's probably a corner of your mind in which there's an unfulfilled wish – that you'd taken up music, or painting, or hang-gliding, or acquired a degree. But of course, now it's too late, and you're too busy, or too old … That unfulfilled part of you may be contributing towards keeping you awake.

You don't have to be brilliantly talented to enjoy singing with a choir, or the pleasure of putting colours on canvas. You don't have to be a genius to enjoy the stimulation and companionship of a creative writing class, or the fun of belonging to an amateur theatrical group. Maybe you feel you've never exercised your brain enough; don't forget the Open University, or studying for A-levels at an evening class or by correspondence.

Even if you don't think you're particularly clever or creative, or your domestic set-up makes it difficult to get out to classes, skills like knitting or crochet, which engage your mind and hands gently, can be very satisfying. Some people find doing jigsaw puzzles immensely soothing.

Growing plants, acquiring a pet, joining a cookery class – there are all kinds of ways in which you can take your mind away from anxiety or loneliness or depression, and focus it on something that gives you pleasure.

This is something you can do all the time, incidentally. So often we move about the world abstractedly, ruminating about the past or the future and missing out on present pleasures. Make a point of noticing what gives you pleasure or lifts your spirits as you go through the day, however small: a child's smile, the colours of nature, the sight of a brilliantly coloured flower-stall – do you pass these things by, or do you take them in and allow them to nourish your spirit?

LIVING IN THE PRESENT

Anxiety and sadness, anger and resentment, are always concerned with either past or future. If you are totally focused in the present moment you *can't* be anxious. So try to take opportunities of living in the present as much as you can.

Put your full attention on whatever you are doing at the time when you're doing it, whether it's working, walking, or washing up. Let your thinking mind off the hook for a few minutes; pause and be aware of your physical body, of your feet on the ground, and your surroundings. If you are out walking, simply look at and experience the sights and sounds, without getting involved in a long train of thought. Gradually you will learn to switch off that over-busy mind and give it and you a rest.

Happiness, the opposite of anxiety and depression, is only ever found in the present moment. We look back with nostalgia, thinking 'If only things had been different!', or forward to achievements we believe will make us feel good; or we believe that someone else could make us happy, if only they would behave differently.

If you remember the real moments of happiness in your life you will know that they don't really depend on other people or events, but on feeling good with yourself. Living in the present helps us to accept ourselves as we are, without judging ourselves by other people's standards. It takes practice, and may not come easily at first, but it's another habit that can be cultivated. And it's a healing habit: one woman totally cured her depression by living in the present, giving up all regrets about the past and fears for the future.

It's also a habit you can take to bed with you. Instead of worrying about whether or when you are going to get to sleep, simply be with yourself in the present moment, regretting nothing, expecting nothing, giving your body and mind permission to let go and rest.

CHAPTER 10

A change of pace

Over the last few years the media have made it very clear that exercise is good for us. For the sake of your sleep you really do need to exercise regularly; the occasional burst won't do much for you. One experiment showed that a single bout of strenuous daytime exercise increased the amount of slow-wave sleep that night in people who were already fit, but had no effect on the sleep of the unfit. On the other hand, research shows that athletes who exercise consistently seem to have more deep, delta sleep than non-exercisers, and when deprived of their exercise their delta sleep diminishes.

If you are physically unable to exercise, don't despair. According to Dr Jim Horne, there is no fall in slow-wave sleep in paraplegics or people obliged to take long periods of bed-rest.* It seems as if the body–mind system adjusts

* James Horne, *Why We Sleep* (Oxford University Press, 1988)

to such situations. But the potentially active body, under-used, will express its dissatisfaction by keeping you awake.

Regular exercise undoubtedly contributes to general health and well-being. For one thing, it tires the body in a healthy way – which is quite different from the tiredness you feel when you've been rushing round getting mentally exhausted, or not rushing round, and getting bored and frustrated.

Exercise is also a wonderful way of clearing the body of the stress hormones that keep so many people awake, anxious or depressed. It can also help to clear your body if you are giving up smoking, alcohol or any other kind of drug. And it's a wonderful way to get over depression or grief. Some people have lifted themselves right out of depression through regular running or jogging. A widowed friend of mine coped with the worst of her bereavement by joining a rambling club and walking for miles every weekend – an excellent recipe for good sleep.

A word of caution: avoid taking exercise late at night, which actually over-stimulates the body. One man who

sought help for insomnia was found to be running for
several miles late every night. The simple answer was
to schedule his exercise earlier in the day. For sleeping
purposes, while a gentle walk round the block to unwind
last thing is fine, the best times for strenuous exercise are
the afternoon and early evening.

WHAT KIND OF EXERCISE?

If you're out of training, don't go in for a sudden
enthuasistic burst and then give up on it; build up slowly
and naturally. Try walking rather than driving or taking
public transport to the station or to work; climb stairs
rather than taking lifts. If you normally spend your lunch
hour in a pub or canteen, try to take twenty to thirty
minutes of that time walking (and I don't mean
shopping).

If you're not geared to exercising, it really is very helpful
to join a class; having a regular commitment to a group

helps to keep you motivated. It's also a good way of making new friends. Have a look at what's available at your local evening institute, adult education or health centre. Competitive sports like tennis, squash and golf can also be beneficial, but not if losing makes you upset or angry. Games are supposed to be enjoyable.

If you're a rusher-round consider taking up a calming form of movement, like T'ai Chi or Yoga. Both will help to balance your energy system, as well as calming mind and body, and both can help you to face life with more tranquillity. Swimming is good, too, with its rhythmic movement and deep breathing; so is walking in the country.

If you are anxious or depressed pick a class with plenty of movement – again, make sure it's enjoyable, not a form of self-punishment. Aerobics, modern and jazz dance, and Medau movement are all cheering and energizing. Any kind of dance is good; some women who've taken up Spanish or Egyptian dancing have found a side benefit in the form of greater self-esteem. Even bopping to the radio or a tape at home can quickly lift your spirits; it's really difficult to be depressed when you're dancing.

For self-esteem, the increasingly popular martial arts are also good. Aikido or judo, for instance, will strengthen both your body and your sense of self.

If you are retired, getting enough exercise will help to keep you healthy and youthful. If you've let yourself go, build up slowly, but add a bit more movement to your day, even if it's just an extra walk round the block. Evening institutes often arrange movement and even yoga classes for the over 60s.

Whatever type you decide on, commit yourself to exercising regularly; build up slowly, and enjoy it.

RELAXATION AND MEDITATION

The onset of normal sleep is a drowsy, relaxed state, a state of peaceful letting go. It should be a state that we drift into naturally, yet in this busy, stressed age, many people have simply lost the art of relaxation, and have to relearn it.

Watching television, going to the cinema, socializing and other off-duty activities all have their place, but they are not really relaxing.

True relaxation involves switching off the active left brain, and also the part of the nervous system that gears us up for action. It reverses the process of building up tension by bringing into play the parasympathetic nervous system, which counteracts the effects of stress, and helps to strengthen the immune system. Regular relaxation can actually alter body chemistry, and deep states can help the brain to produce endorphins, hormones that have been called 'the body's own morphine', which have the effects of lifting the mood and relieving pain.

Meditation has many similar effects. Though relaxation is aimed chiefly at the body, and meditation at the mind and spirit, both slow down and rebalance the body–mind system. Many people who meditate regularly find they need less sleep than before, because during their meditation periods they are giving their systems deep rest. Both meditation and relaxation require us, and also enable us, to let go of worry and tension and focus on the present moment.

Some people are quite scared of letting go; they feel they must hang on and stay in control. This is partly because many of us have been brought up with the idea that 'doing nothing' is a waste of precious time, possibly even sinful; partly because of a not always conscious fear that something terrible will happen if we let go. The most vivid example of this I ever saw was on a plane journey with a friend who was scared of flying: she sat rigid in her seat clutching the armrests, and I suddenly realized that *she was actually trying to hold the plane up.*

Letting go is a normal part of life's rhythm; hanging on to control builds up physical tensions which go to bed with you. A tense mind is less able to solve problems than a relaxed one: if you learn to relax you will find that it will not make you less efficient, but better able to cope, and with more control over your waking and sleeping patterns.

In 1985 a small study was carried out by the Sleep Laboratory at Leeds University, with a group of airline pilots. Pilots have such irregular hours and routines that they often have to take sleeping pills to get their rest, a far from ideal situation. Ten pilots were taught a mixture of muscle relaxation and mental meditational techniques, which enabled them to get to sleep whenever they needed to, in unusual environments, even on long taxi-rides. Eight months later, seven of them were still using these techniques; of the remaining three, one had been practising his own form of meditation before the study.

Most people in these tense days could benefit from regular relaxation or meditation. Build it into your day: give yourself a space to practise for 20 minutes at least once a day.

LEARNING TO RELAX

Although there are some excellent books on relaxation, if you are under severe tension there is nothing to beat personal tuition, in a group or class where you can get individual attention.

If you want to make a start on your own, choose a time and a place where you will be peaceful and undisturbed. Tell yourself that you are going to devote the next 20 minutes to completely letting go. (The aeroplane won't fall down!) Sit comfortably with your back supported and your feet flat on the floor, your hands loose in your lap and your eyes closed. Or lie down, with your head and knees supported by cushions. There are several relaxation techniques favoured by experts. Here are two.

Progressive relaxation consists of alternately tensing and relaxing all the muscles in your body, from toe to head, or head to toe, in turn. Take it slowly. When you've been through all the muscles, notice if there are any tense spots left, and let them go. The jaw is often a tension-site; clench it and then let it drop. Make sure your tongue is relaxed too. Then enjoy the sense of relaxation until your 20 minutes are up. Come out of it slowly; if you jump up you may find yourself slightly giddy.

Another method is to start sitting or lying, stretch the whole body, and let it go, like a cat. Then simply sense that waves of relaxation are flowing through your body as you breathe in, while more and more tension is leaving you with every out-breath.

Relaxation can be aided by using mental imagery; as you let go physically, imagine that you are floating on a cloud or on a lilo on a sun-lit sea; or that you are a cat, totally relaxed and oblivious of your surroundings; or a heavy sackful of sand; or a balloon floating in a blue sky. (Images of both lightness and heaviness seem to aid relaxation equally well.)

Cassette tapes can also help you learn to relax on your own; there are a number of good ones on the market. Don't, however, become dependent on one tape. What you are aiming for is the ability to relax whenever you want to – not just at special relaxation times.

MEDITATION TECHNIQUES

These take you into a relaxed state through the mind. Their object is to reach a state of inner peace by quietening mental chatter, often by focusing on a word, sound, or object. Again, I feel it's important that meditation should be taught personally or in a group; the inexperienced meditator often strains to concentrate, and guidance may be needed in letting go.

If you want to try if for yourself, start with five or ten minutes at a time. Sit as for the relaxation exercise above, making sure you won't be disturbed. Then try one of the following:

Gently repeat mentally a single word, for example 'harmony'. Rest your attention on this word without straining. Every time you find your mind wandering, bring it back to the word.

Put your attention on your breathing, simply being aware of it without trying to change it. It can help you to concentrate if you count from one to ten as you do so, counting 'one-and', 'two-and' and so on with each in-out breath. If you lose count, return to 'one'.

At the end of any relaxation or meditation exercise, don't leap back into activity, but come out slowly and gently, bringing some of that inner peace into the rest of your life.

Research shows that several relaxation techniques can be beneficial for insomniacs, including progressive relaxation, relaxation-meditation, biofeedback assisted meditation and autogenic training. Whatever method is used, it needs to be practised regularly, both with an instructor and at home.

Some people find it difficult to relax because they simply don't know what relaxation feels like. Many of the natural therapies can help you to regain that experience, particularly hands-on treatments like the Alexander Technique, massage, sacral-cranial therapy and spiritual healing. Some forms of exercise are also very relaxing; Yoga includes techniques for whole-body relaxation and meditation, while T'ai Chi has been described as meditation in movement.

Breathing

Correct breathing is important in both relaxation and meditation. As body and mind slow down, so does the breath; conversely, slowing and deepening your breathing automatically makes you calmer. However, when we are tense we tend to breathe fast and shallowly, high up in the chest, which makes it very hard to relax. Some chronically tense people hyper-ventilate; that is, they over-breathe all the time, which keeps them in a permanent state of anxiety. Hyperventilation also prevents sufficient oxygen reaching the brain and can have other unpleasant side effects like migraines, dizziness, nausea and palpitations.

Learning to breathe naturally helps you to keep calm. Try this: lie on the floor with a cushion or book under your head. Put a heavy-ish object (a large book or a beanbag) on your midriff, between your abdomen and lower ribs. As you breathe in and out, the object should rise and fall; if it doesn't, you are breathing too high up in the chest.

Using the weight as a guide, you can retrain yourself to breathe diaphragmatically: full breathing should expand your diaphragm, lower ribs, and abdomen. Don't *force* yourself to breathe deeply; simply be aware of how you are breathing now. Then think of your ribs and lungs expanding and contracting, and allow your breath to become deeper, slower and calmer. Think of your ribs expanding sideways as well as up and down. If you practise this for a few minutes every day, you will acquire the habit of calmer, relaxing breathing when you get to bed at night.

Another sign of anxiety is holding your breath. A good exercise when you feel yourself tensing up during the day is to consciously breathe out, at the same time letting the tension flow away from your neck, shoulders and arms. Practise this in situations which would normally make you uptight: in traffic jams and queues, or waiting to be put through on the telephone. As it starts to become a habitual response, you can use these occasions as opportunities for relaxation instead of anxiety, irritation or anger.

A good method of getting back in touch with your body and breathing pattern is the Alexander Technique, which (among its other benefits) helps to free tensions locked into the back and rib-cage. Osteopathy and chiropractic can also help to free tight chest muscles, enabling you to breathe more fully. Yoga, too, lays much stress on breathing; one very simple exercise is to breathe in to the count of six, hold your breath to the count of six, breathe out to the count of six, and then either breathe in again or hold the outbreath for six, before resuming the cycle. It is very calming.

CHAPTER II

Food and other habits

It's impossible to get a really healthy balance in life without including nutrition. Food and drink have a direct chemical influence on our bodies, nervous system and moods. Over-indulgence in junk food, coffee or alcohol – all of which often accompany a stressed lifestyle – affects your well-being, simultaneously over-stimulating the adrenal glands and nervous system and depleting the body of essential vitamins and minerals. In addition, some foods are more stimulating and some more sedative in their own right.

We get many contradictory messages these days about what's good for us and what isn't. And of course individual needs differ; while more and more people are becoming vegetarian, for instance, there are others whose systems really seem to need meat. If you're any doubt, consult a naturopath or nutritionist about your needs.

Meanwhile, here are some general guidelines which hold good for everyone who wants to sleep better.

Foods and drinks to go for:

Plenty of fresh fruit and salads, dried fruits, green and root vegetables, *live* yogurt (if it suits you), whole grains (brown rice, oats, wholemeal bread and flour), pulses (lentils and dried beans), fish and free-range chicken rather than red meats, and a moderate amount of fats, eggs, cheese and dairy products. Among these foods, the more stimulating are raw vegetables, salads and fruits; so naturopaths recommend fruit and/or dried fruit with breakfast and a large raw salad with lunch.

Root vegetables are believed to be more sedative than those growing above ground; also sedative are the unrefined carbohydrates – potatoes, and wholegrain bread, pasta and rice, so these are best eaten with the evening meal.

Many foods, when combined with carbohydrates, lead to the production of an amino-acid called tryptophan, the main building block for serotonin, a neurochemical which is produced as a precursor to sleep. They include milk, eggs, meat, nuts, fish, hard cheeses, bananas and pulses.

Drink herbal teas, spring water and pure fruit juices, or some of the non-caffeinated drinks you can buy in health food stores, such as dandelion coffee (made from the dried root rather than powder), or cereal drinks like Barley Cup and Pionier.

FOODS AND DRINKS TO AVOID:

Sugar (including cakes, chocolate, biscuits etc.)

Refined carbohydrates (white flour and sugar), which fill you up and overwork the digestive system without giving your body any real fuel.

Processed foods. We have been made aware of the dangers of chemical additives, especially to the allergy-prone, but many processed foods still contain additives to which some people have an adverse reaction without always realizing it. In particular, tartrazine (E102) and monosodium glutamate can upset people's sleeping patterns, especially if eaten in the evening.

High-fat foods also put a strain on the digestive system when eaten in the evening – so there may be some truth in the suggestion that cheese can give you bad dreams!

Caffeine, found not just in coffee, but in tea, colas, and chocolate, doesn't only affect you late at night. It can contribute to nervousness and depression at any time.

Excess salt raises the blood pressure and puts the body into overdrive.

THE TIMING OF MEALS

Far less well publicized than what we eat is the importance of *when* we eat. The old adage, 'breakfast like a king, lunch like a lord and dine like a pauper', is supported by naturopaths and other natural practitioners, who recommend a hearty breakfast, a moderate lunch, and a light supper, eaten if possible no later than 6 p.m.

There are very good biological reasons for this: the human digestive system functions best in the morning, when it produces a good supply of enzymes for the quick and efficient absorption of nutrients. The digestive process gets slower throughout the day, really starting to slow down around 6 p.m.; by nine it is very sluggish indeed.

You may *feel* sleepy after a heavy meal, because the blood goes from the head to the stomach, but still find it difficult to get to sleep because your body has been given an extra hard task when it should be resting – *you* wouldn't like to start work at bedtime either! In addition, digestion takes place most efficiently when the body is upright.

Although people's body clocks differ, this slowing down of digestion seems to be true for everyone. This means that food eaten late in the evening is liable to remain in the stomach half-digested and putrefying all night, affecting both sleep and our enthusiasm for breakfast in the morning. In some cases it can actually cause a build-up of toxins, leading to ill-health.

If you habitually sleep badly, a large breakfast may well be the last thing you feel like in the morning. But remember that you are now changing your habits to encourage your body to relax and sleep; how you start the day will affect how you end it. If you try for a three-week period having a good lunch and an early, light supper, you'll soon find yourself much keener on breakfast.

A hearty and healthy breakfast could include porridge, or an oat-based muesli (oats are excellent nerve strengtheners) with yoghurt and dried or fresh fruit, and/or wholemeal toast with honey, or cheese if you like it. No more than three eggs (preferably free-range) should be eaten per week.

Unfortunately, our social system is not geared to our body clocks and for the rest of the day you may have to do some adaptation. The lordly lunch accompanied by a large salad may not be available where you work, and if you have a long journey home, the early, light supper may present difficulties. Experiment with packed lunches; raw carrots, celery and apples need scarcely any preparation. If possible, finish your evening meal by 8 p.m. at the latest.

If you are going straight from work to an evening class,

have your hot meal at lunchtime and a sandwich or baked potato before the class. And if you're invited out for a late, delicious dinner – keep the portions down (and the alcohol), relax and enjoy it! Eating *happily* is possibly as important as what you eat.

ALLERGIES AND SENSITIVITIES

If you suffer severely from a food allergy you will probably already be aware of it. But degrees of allergic reaction vary; some people are sensitive to particular foods without having an out-and-out allergy. Their degree of sensitivity can also vary, with reactions worse at particularly stressful times and unnoticeable at others. The substances most commonly causing allergic reactions or intolerance are wheat, eggs, dairy products, sugar and caffeine, as well as certain chemicals and additives.

Very often, people are unaware that something they've been enjoying for years is affecting them badly. This is a common phenomenon known as a masked allergy, when sufferers are actually addicted to the substance that is doing them harm.

It's worth observing your reactions to foods and drinks, particularly those you crave for or consume every day. If you notice that you regularly feel extra hyped up or depressed after any of these, try cutting them out of your diet for a week or two and see whether this makes a difference. If you are suffering from a masked allergy you may get slight withdrawal symptoms; people giving up caffeine, for instance, sometimes experience headaches and fuzziness for a few days. If this happens to you, tell yourself it's actually a good sign, showing that your system is cleansing itself of something that was doing it harm. Drink plenty of spring water to help it along.

SUPPLEMENTS

Views on the value of vitamin and mineral supplements
vary wildly, particularly between orthodox medical doctors
and supplement-minded practitioners. The general
orthodox view is that so long as you eat a healthy,
balanced diet, you don't need anything extra. However,
natural therapists point out that so much of our food
is de-natured by things like pesticides, pollution and
preservatives that most people's vitamin and mineral
intake needs topping up. This is certainly so when
someone is under stress, as is likely to be the case with
insomniacs.

At the same time, supplements are only useful when
they supply what you personally are short of. Taking more
of a vitamin or mineral than you actually need is wasteful,
and can in some cases be harmful; in others, taking
supplements will have no effect if for some reason your
body is not absorbing them. On top of this, there is an
increasingly bewildering array in health food shops of not

only vitamins and herbal remedies but amino-acids and unusual minerals. Advice from a homoeopath, naturopath, nutritionist, or kinesiologist (see Chapter 14) can help you to sort out your personal needs, and may save you a lot of expense on unnecessary, useless, or incompletely researched supplements.

In general, however, it can be both helpful and safe to take a good combined vitamin and mineral pill daily. If you are highly stressed you can safely take daily an extra 1000mg of Vitamin C (with bioflavonoids) and 25mg B6 (which helps the body make use of tryptophan); this should be accompanied by a B-complex tablet. If you smoke, you need extra amounts of both B and C since nicotine leaches these vitamins, as well as some minerals, from the system.

The mineral calcium is widely recommended for nerves and anxiety; a naturopath recommends taking 200mg daily in the form of Dolomite tablets, which contain natural calcium combined with magnesium, another stress reducer which also helps the body to absorb the calcium.

Zinc can also be useful, particularly if you are depressed; since this comes in many varieties, consult your health food shop owner or natural health practitioner before buying.

A WORD ABOUT ALCOHOL

It's true that a small amount of alcohol is a relaxant, and can blur the edges of anxiety. But there are both disadvantages and risks in the alcoholic night-cap. Alcohol is a drug; it's possible for one glass to turn into two, or more … and before you know it you have developed a dependency. And even if it helps you to get off to sleep initially, alcohol can actually *cause* insomnia. To digest it, your liver and kidneys have to work extra hard, and your body has to provide extra adrenalin – which is, of course, a stimulant. It has been found that after alcohol intake, sleep is more disturbed with more awakenings; alcohol also reduces REM sleep.

Drinking large amounts of alcohol regularly can lead to alcohol addiction – alcoholism, in other words – which affects your body, your work, and your relationships, and your sleep.

So, ideally, stick to no more than a glass or two of wine, two or three days a week; you'll feel better for it all round. If you feel deprived on non-alcohol days, boost your morale by telling yourself you're giving your body – especially your hard-working liver – a nice rest!

SMOKING

Nicotine is also a stimulant, which can exacerbate sleeplessness, particularly as you grow older. Non-insomniac smokers have been found to take longer to go to sleep than non-smokers and wake up more often during the night. In a trial at Pennsylvania State University, when eight heavy smokers gave up abruptly, the time they took to get to sleep dropped from an average 52 minutes to 18 on the first two nights, and this pattern continued in four of them who continued without smoking for two weeks.

Initially, giving up may cause a short-term increase in tension, and if you are under a lot of stress at the moment this may not be the best time to stop. But do cut down, especially in the evenings, and try not to smoke during the last hour before going to bed. One way of cutting down is to tell yourself, every time you reach for a cigarette, that you'll have it later.

If you make a real commitment to stop, this could obviously improve your sleep quite rapidly. You can get many forms of help and support from a number of natural therapies which will help to calm your nervous system and support you during the withdrawal phase. These include a choice of acupuncture, homoeopathy, herbalism, hypnotherapy, kinesiology, and relaxation.

CHAPTER 12

Bedtime

The hour or two leading up to bedtime should be a time of slowly winding-down, letting go of the day and its busyness. If you need to have a family discussion (or worse), get it over early, and leave matters as resolved as they can be. Write down anything unresolved, and make a definite appointment with yourself and anyone else involved to continue it another time, not in bed.

The same goes for anything else that might be worrying you. Early in the evening, write it down, write down any decisions you have made about dealing with it, and then say goodbye to it for today. *You have done all you can.*

Keep your bedtime as regular as possible; while you are retraining your body–mind system, late nights are not a good idea. Although scientifically it's not been proven that the hours before midnight are best for sleep, some natural practitioners believe that they are. Round about ten p.m.

our body clocks begin to slow down and gear themselves for sleep.

Try to observe your own natural rhythm, and don't stay up beyond the time when you naturally feel sleepy, even if that means forgoing the end of an interesting TV programme. Some experts recommend that you don't watch television during the hours before bedtime, since the flickering image can stimulate the nervous system. However, I think this must depend on both the person and the programme. A cheering or funny programme may help you go to bed in a good mood. But don't fall asleep while you're watching it: you'll have to wake up again in order to go to bed – very confusing to your body clock, which then makes it hard to get off again.

The same goes for reading in bed. While the stimulus-control programme described in Chapter 2 says the bedroom is only for sleep, some people do find reading in bed a good way to switch their mind away from the worries of the day. This again must be your own choice. But don't waver between systems: if you've chosen to adopt the stimulus-control programme, stick to it for the whole three weeks.

BEDTIME DRINKS

A hot bedtime drink can be soothing and comforting – but bear in mind that it will reach your bladder in the small hours. This might seem obvious, but I've come across more than one elderly person complaining of having to get up to go to the bathroom, without connecting it with their late-night cup of tea! As we get older our kidneys become more active during the night, so the amount an elderly person can comfortably drink before bed will be less than in his or her younger days. If your bladder is a problem, try having your bedtime drink no later than an hour before bedtime.

The tradition of having a hot milky drink at bedtime is probably based on the fact that milk contains both tryptophan and calcium, which is a muscle relaxant and soothing to the nervous system. A cup of hot milk accompanied by a couple of Dolomite tablets (containing calcium and magnesium) can help you get off to sleep, and helps some sufferers from restless legs.

Not all proprietary milky drinks are actually good for sleep; chocolate, for instance, has a high caffeine content. Best is plain hot milk, with maybe a teaspoon of honey, or a malted milk like Horlicks. A sprinkling of grated nutmeg on top is also sleep inducing. If your sleeplessness is related to indigestion, Slippery Elm makes a soothing drink.

Some people find milk hard to digest, and as it is a food in its own right dietary purists would not recommend it last thing at night. This also applies to late night snacks, of course. Some people recommend eating a snack of foods containing tryptophan last thing at night – a bowl of cereal, a banana, or a lettuce sandwich for instance. As discussed in the last chapter, this is the time when the body should be geared for sleep, not for digesting food – and food eaten last thing is more likely to end up as stored fat.

However, this is a choice you must make for yourself: if a late-night snack suits you and helps you sleep, that may be the most important factor while you recover your sleep pattern.

Some people find cider vinegar and honey helps them to sleep; the mixture contains a good supply of trace elements including calcium. Take a teaspoonful of each in a small cup of boiling water.

A very pleasant late-night drink is Norfolk Punch, a non-alcoholic blend of herbs and spices found in health food shops and recommended as a relaxant. Some people find that it loses its efficacy if drunk every night; have it as a treat after a particularly fraught day.

HERBAL DRINKS

Herb teas are becoming increasingly popular as replacements for caffeine-containing drinks. There is a good variety of herbal tea-bags in the shops, some of them specially blended to help you relax or sleep. They are quite expensive; it's cheaper to buy loose herbs from a herbalist or health food shop and experiment with single herbs or mixtures. Herbs can lose their efficacy over time, so buy them in small quantities, keep them in air-tight jars, and use them promptly.

HERBAL INFUSIONS

Herbal infusions are slightly stronger than teas, and can be taken medicinally three times a day. You can make up an infusion of one or more herbs, using 1–2 heaped teaspoonfuls of dried leaves or flowers to a cup of water. Use a herbal infuser or small teapot, and pour the water onto the herbs when just on the boil. Leave to stand, covered, for at least 5–10 minutes before drinking, up to 20 minutes if you are taking them medicinally.

Camomile is one of the best-known herbs for calming the nerves, and for settling the digestion. It is said to have cumulative effects, becoming more effective over a period of time. However, some people find the flavour rather bland, and it has the disadvantage of being mildly diuretic.

Lime-flower (linden) makes a very effective and pleasant flavoured night-cap and is good for headaches, nervous tension and restlessness. The herbalist Michael McIntyre, co-author of *The Complete New Herbal** told me that when he lived in France hyperactive children would be taken out to have tea under the lime trees in summer, because of their calming effect. And it didn't only calm children. 'The bees were narcotized,' he said. 'You'd see them lying there glugging gently because they'd had a bit too much lime flower while taking the nectar!' (A nice image to go to bed with!)

Scullcap is a tonic as well as a sedative, high in magnesium and calcium, which help to strengthen the nervous system. It is not always easy to obtain, and what is often sold as scullcap is another herb called teucrium

* Richard Mabey (ed.), *The Complete New Herbal*, (Elm Tree Books, 1988)

(wood sage). So get the genuine article, *Scutellaria lateriflora*, from a reputable herbalist.

Passiflora (passion flower) is another good soporific, a constituent of many herbal sleeping pills.

Valerian root is well-known as a sedative. It tastes like old socks (and smells worse) but a proportion of it can be mixed with more pleasant-flavoured herbs. Valerian has a more 'druggy' effect than most herbs, and some people find it gives them headaches if drunk in large quantities; so (unless prescribed by a herbalist) don't take it consecutively for more than a week or two.

Hawthorn flowers are good for people who don't sleep because they have heart palpitations.

Mint is good for soothing the digestion.

Lemon balm and vervain are good for depression.

BATH-TIME

Wash off any remaining stresses of the day by having a bath before bed, and make it sleep-inducing with the help of herbal or aromatherapy preparations. Enjoy your bath as a relaxing treatment; make it warm but not too hot, and give yourself time to soak in the oils or herbs so that you get the full, soothing benefit.

Suitable aromatherapy oils include lavender (used regularly it has the advantage of boosting your immune system, but go easy on it if you are pregnant), camomile and orange blossom (both rather expensive), meadowsweet, geranium and hops. Use no more than four to six drops of oil or oils altogether, using the smaller amount if your skin is very sensitive. Agitate the water so that the oil spreads evenly and reaches your whole body. Allow yourself time to soak, relax and absorb the oil both through your skin and by inhaling the vapour.

Herbs can also be used in the bath by making an extra strong infusion, strained and poured into your bath water.

Lime-flowers are good; so are hops: pour a cup of boiling water over three crushed heads and steep, covered, for ten minutes. You can also use lavender, or a mixture of herbs: fill a muslin bag with the heads and tie it to the hot tap, so that the hot water runs through it. Before getting into the bath, add a strained infusion of the same herbs.

Herbal baths are also soothing for babies. Michael McIntyre says: 'Camomile herb is a very suitable way to get your baby to sleep. You can give your baby a camomile bath. Make a strong tea using an ounce to two pints of water, strain it, and add it to the water in the baby-bath.' And Barbara Griggs quotes the French herbalist Maurice Messegué who 'recalls being put in a bath of Lime Flowers and Leaves as a child when he couldn't sleep – with magical results …'*

* Barbara Griggs, *The Home Herbal: A Handbook of Simple Remedies,* (Jill Norman and Hobhouse, 1982)

GOING TO BED

After your bath, if you have a partner who is willing
to gently massage your neck and shoulders or feet, do
encourage this. If you're on your own, gently massage
the bits you can reach, and do some gentle stretching and
yawning before you get into bed.

Go to bed in cotton night-wear rather than artificial
fibre. Some people find it helpful to put a few drops of an
essential oil on the pillow – lavender is particularly good.
But don't put the drops where your face will come into
direct contact with them; undiluted essential oils are quite
powerful and can cause skin reactions.

Some people find it helpful just before or just after
getting into bed to review the day, and then say a firm
goodbye to it. Try it: note particularly the things you have
enjoyed, however small, and say thank you for them.

Once in bed, relax and let go. Allow your body to be
as comfortable as possible, and know that your mind will
soon be taking you into sleep. Don't *try* to get to sleep;

rather, think of sleep as a friend for whom you have made all the right preparations, and who will arrive in his own good time. Remember that the normal person takes 15–20 minutes to get to sleep, so there's no rush. Only a few happy souls hit sleep when their heads hit the pillow.

If you are still awake after 20 minutes, you have a choice. The stimulus control programme recommends that you get up and *do* something, in a different room. Have a hot drink, or read, or write a letter, until you feel sleepy enough to return to bed. The same rule applies if you wake up in the middle of the night.

The alternative is to stay in bed, but allowing yourself to think of pleasant things. Don't lie there worrying or brooding.

Whichever system you opt for, commit yourself to it for at least three weeks.

NIGHT THOUGHTS

If your body is relaxed but your mind still active, either before going to sleep or after waking up in the small hours, you can train yourself not to focus on anxiety and worry by concentrating on something else.

One method is to play mental games which will keep your mind occupied and possibly rather bored until you drop off. These include things like counting backwards from 100–1, or listing in alphabetical order the names of your friends, or countries, or flowers. You could consider learning a verse or two of a poem before turning in and reciting it to yourself in bed. Or just pick a harmonious line of poetry, and mentally repeat it to yourself over and over.

Listening to the radio has been the resort of many insomniacs, as you will probably have discovered for yourself, but it has the disadvantage that if there's a really interesting programme, you may stay awake to hear it to the end.

If worrying thoughts come into your head, let them go, with the knowledge that you will deal with them at the proper time. As you breathe in, think of peace, tranquillity, calmness entering your system; breathe the worry away.

Another way of dealing with negative or anxious thoughts is not to fight them, but to listen to them in a detached manner as if they were a rather boring radio programme, without trying to find solutions to them.

Mind-games can include images that help to activate the alpha waves that precede sleep: you could take yourself on an imaginary or remembered walk in the country or by the sea. Or take yourself through a film you have really enjoyed.

The more pleasant your thoughts, the more likely you are to relax and go off to sleep. Remember the image of your mind energy: negative thoughts press down on you, while happy ones lift depression away from you. So do thoughts that are not focused on yourself.

I discovered accidentally one wakeful night that praying for other people sent me off in no time. Obviously, the purpose of prayer is not to send you to sleep, nor do I assume that everyone believes in prayer. But if you find your mind returning to your own problems, it may help you to switch your attention to a friend or friends who would benefit from a healing thought from you. If they are ill, don't focus on their illness, but visualize them well and happy, or imagine a stream of healing white or gold light going from your heart to surround them. If you don't visualize clearly, this is not important: simply send them well-wishing thoughts.

If someone pops into your mind who has hurt, insulted, irritated or angered you, send them a healing thought too – they probably need it.

And if you're one of those people who lies awake worrying about the environment, try sending healing thoughts to the planet, to animals, trees and nature, which will do both you and the environment much more good than if you lie there worrying about it.

CHAPTER 13

How natural therapies can help

There is an ever-increasing variety of natural therapies available today, some complementary to orthodox medicine and some alternative; those most appropriate to sleeplessness are described in the next chapter. What they have in common is the principle that we all have our own powers of self-healing. They aim to remove blockages to health by restoring harmony and balance, rather than zapping symptoms with drugs which can actually deplete the patient's life force. While their methods vary, they work on the basis that body, mind and emotions are a single, interdependent unit, and that for a healthy system, all three need to be attended to.

As well as curing or relieving medical problems, natural therapies can help you to relax, and can relieve pain and anxiety. Many practitioners are also good counsellors who will provide emotional support to deal with the causes of your insomnia, or with withdrawal from tranquillizers or sleeping pills.

By contrast with conventional medicine, practitioners of natural medicines treat the person rather than the disease, which can involve a multiplicity of approaches, even within the same disciplines. They take into account the patient's personality and lifestyle, recognizing that people vary in their responses to the same treatment. (To be fair to doctors, an increasing number nowadays also aim to treat patients in this holistic way.)

Another difference with conventional medicine is the speed at which treatments work. We have become used to a course of antibiotics, for instance, taking effect very speedily (and there are certainly emergency occasions when antibiotics are very useful). But antibiotics work by suppressing symptoms; natural medicines treat the mind and body which have become sufficiently depleted for bacteria or viruses to flourish, and symptoms are regarded as the body's efforts to defend itself.

This means that restoring health to the whole person

can take time. In addition, cure often involves what's known as a healing crisis, when symptoms temporarily worsen as the body starts fighting back. So don't be disappointed if results aren't instant; give whatever therapy you choose at least a couple of months to see how it's affecting you. A good practitioner will be happy to discuss your progress with you after the first few visits, and may then be able to give you an idea of how long treatment will take.

As far as insomnia is concerned, however, since natural treatments can be very relaxing, this is often one of the first symptoms to go.

CHOOSING A THERAPY

The plethora of possible therapies can be quite confusing to the new patient. In addition, most individual therapies are taught at a number of different training schools, which often vary in their emphasis and approach. What is important is to find both a therapy and a practitioner that suit you personally. Often the qualities of the practitioner as a person are at least as important as the techniques he or she uses.

The therapies described in the following pages can all be helpful for emotional stress, physical tension and pain, as well as insomnia. If touch is lacking in your life, you might receive particular benefit from a hands-on treatment like osteopathy, chiropractic, aromatherapy, or massage. If you feel taking medication is important or necessary, try homoeopathy or medical herbalism.

Before embarking on a course of treatment it's worth checking out what the practitioner has to offer in addition to any specialization. Some train in more than one discipline, and can advise you on diet or nutritional supplements, or combine treatments like osteopathy and acupuncture.

You may find your practitioner using unusual means of diagnosis: some are trained in iridology, diagnosis through the iris of the eye, which reflects the state of the body:

variations in the colour, dark or light spots and so on can indicate organic or functional weaknesses and nutritional deficiencies. Some use kinesiology techniques (see page 148) to test imbalances and nutritional needs; some use dowsing with a pendulum. Some are highly intuitive and can tell a lot about a patient simply by looking at them or touching them.

Assuming your GP is open minded, it's as well to let him or her know that you are seeking additional treatment. Doctors today are conscious of the possible side-effects of tranquillizers and sleeping pills; they don't want patients to become addicted, and many of them recognize the value of alternative forms of reducing anxiety.

However, if you are already taking medication you should discuss this with both your doctor and the natural practitioner you have chosen. Some forms of natural medicine really are alternative rather than complementary to conventional medicine; some herbal medicines, for example, may not be compatible with medical drugs, and the effect of some homoeopathic remedies can be counteracted by drugs like steroids. So you should talk to your doctor before making any changes in or adding to what he or she has already prescribed.

CHAPTER 14

The therapies

ACUPUNCTURE

Acupuncture can be an effective treatment for insomnia, by restoring balance and harmony to the patient's energy system. Return to normal sleep may take several sessions, but some people feel extremely relaxed immediately after or even during a treatment. It can relieve emotional as well as physical pain, calming anxiety and lifting depression. Regarded by most doctors with scepticism only 20 years ago, it is the most widely used complementary therapy within the medical profession, practised by a number of GPs, and increasingly in hospital pain clinics.

This ancient Chinese technique is based on the theory that health depends on a harmonious flow of energy, or life force, called *qi* (pronounced *chee*). *Qi* flows through the body via energy channels called meridians; the twelve main meridians are connected with and named after a physical organ – the heart, lungs, liver, kidneys, and so on – each of which can be affected by a specific emotion. For example, fear affects the kidneys and anger the liver, together with their relevant meridians. Insomnia is often found to relate to a disruption in the energy flow of the heart meridian, which can be caused by shock, or even by excessive joy.

Too much or too little energy in one or more meridians can give rise to both mental and physical symptoms. Diagnosis therefore focuses on the individual's state of energy rather than specific diseases. Traditional methods include taking a full history, observing the patient's skin colour and possibly tongue, and noting which parts of the body are extra hot or cold. The strength of the meridians is checked through twelve pulses found in the wrists. Over- or under-activity in a meridian can be caused by dietary, physical or emotional factors – often a combination of these – and the acupuncturist's aim is to restore health by restoring the balance. Progress is usually slow and steady, but treatment can sometimes have dramatic effects in releasing traumatic memories, and a few acupuncturists combine their treatment with psychotherapy.

Along the meridians lie hundreds of acupuncture points, tiny gateways into the energy flow, whose Chinese names often indicate their function. Treatment consists of stimulating or sedating the meridians to restore the energy balance, by inserting very fine steel needles into the appropriate points. Whether this is painful or not depends both on the practitioner's touch and the patient's sensitivity. Points that need treatment are usually tender to the touch, and may be slightly painful when the needle is first inserted; as the balance is restored, the pain lessens. Usually only a few points are treated in any one session. The needles may be left in place for 10 to 20 minutes, and the acupuncturist may twiddle them from time to time.

For insomnia, the acupuncturist may well treat points on the heart meridian, including *Shenmen* ('gate of the spirit'), an important point on the wrist, which is also often used for depression. In traditional Chinese terms the heart is said to be the seat of the mind or spirit, and sleeplessness is caused by the spirit 'rampaging'. In more orthodox terms, treating the heart meridian takes the pressure off the nerves to the heart, which may be over-stimulated.

Acupuncture can be extremely useful in reducing withdrawal symptoms from tranquillizers, sleeping pills and other drugs including nicotine. Research on heroin addicts in Hong Kong has shown that treatment increases the brain's output of endorphins, reducing pain and lifting the mood. It also stimulates the excretion of drugs from the system. Some acupuncturists prefer patients to come off their pills before starting treatment, since the drugs may counteract the effects of acupuncture.

THE ALEXANDER TECHNIQUE

The Alexander Technique can help you sleep better by creating greater physical and mental harmony, enabling you to go through life with less strain. It is a way of learning how to use your body as it was meant to be used – easily, effortlessly, and without tension.

The Technique was developed in the 1920s by an Australian actor, Frederick Matthias Alexander. Specializing in one-man shows, he was plagued by recurring hoarseness and breathing problems which prevented him from performing. When medical specialists could find nothing wrong with his throat, Alexander decided that there must be something wrong with the way he was using it. He studied himself with the help of mirrors and realized that his voice was being affected by the way he held his head and neck, which in turn related to the tensions in his body.

Over the years he taught himself new habits, not only solving his voice problem but discovering a new mental power and energy. He began teaching his technique to private individuals, including actors: today it is taught at several training schools in Britain, and is very popular among performers of all kinds, who are probably more aware of their bodies than the rest of us.

Small children know instinctively how to hold themselves correctly, but are soon thrown out of balance from schooldays onwards by things like badly designed school desks and too much sedentary work, as well as the stresses of modern living. Emotions are also reflected in the body; rounded shoulders can develop as a fear response to an over-critical or bullying parent, while over-anxiety can produce a head that thrusts forward instead of balancing easily on top of the spine. These muscular postures tend to become fixed, perpetuating the attitudes of mind they reflect.

Lessons usually last 30 to 45 minutes, during which the teacher helps you gradually to adjust the way you stand, sit and walk, using his or her hands to show the body how it should be, and gently guiding your muscles into new habits. It takes time for habits to be changed, and initially you may need to see a teacher once or twice a week; this is gradually tailed off, so that in time you will only need a lesson every month or two. During this re-education process, tensions are released, the stance becomes more natural, the ribs open up so that you breathe more naturally and deeply, and very often back and neck problems are relieved. As the client becomes more self-aware, he or she is able to go through daily life with less stress.

Despite its gentleness, the technique can bring about profound changes not only in the body but in the mind, partly through the letting-go of old tensions, and partly through its focus on the present moment. This can result in a new, freer way of responding to stress, anxiety, decision-making and so on. For insomniacs, learning to adopt a different, more flowing attitude to daily activities can be extremely beneficial.

AROMATHERAPY

Aromatherapy must be one of the most delicious ways of treating insomnia. It consists of massage using essential plant oils in a vegetable oil base, and is a wonderful way to experience deep relaxation, excellent for tension and stress-related conditions.

It is more than a pleasant experience, however. The essential oils are distilled from the flowers, leaves or roots of plants with specific curative properties. Their volatile elements are absorbed through the skin into the bloodstream, and into both the body and brain through the membranes at the back of the nose. They can affect the organs and glands within the body, and have a direct effect on mood, since they reach the parts of the brain controlling the emotions. So there are oils that can simultaneously calm you, clear your brain, and lift depression, as well as healing your physical body.

These days aromatherapy is used in some hospitals and hospices, largely at the instigation of nurses, who recognize the value of healing touch. Within the medical context it does not replace drugs, but it does enhance their effect so that smaller doses can be prescribed.*

A qualified aromatherapist will first take clients through a questionnaire to check on their medical history and specific needs, looking in the case of insomnia for its emotional and physical causes before choosing what combination of oils to use. One of the beauties of aromatherapy is that each oil has several properties, so that you can be treated on several levels at once.

The treatment itself can take up to an hour, sometimes longer, and usually the whole body will be massaged. Some people find themselves going to sleep on the massage table; some find that in this relaxed state they can talk out their problems with the therapist. And because scents can trigger the emotions and the memory, clients may find themselves experiencing an emotional release during or

* Helen Passant, 'A Holistic Approach in the Ward', *Nursing Times* (24–30 January 1990)

after a treatment. 'You release the tensions, and also bring out things that people may have buried,' says aromatherapist Tricia Donà-Hooker. 'When people allow things to come up in them, they can be recognized and dealt with.'

Aromatherapists may well be able to help you come off sleeping pills or tranquillizers, using oils that can both calm you and cleanse your system of the drugs; like other natural therapists they will want you to get your doctor's agreement first.

The choice of oils will depend on the individual's physical and mental state. In *Aromatherapy for Everyone** Robert Tisserand describes how he helped an elderly widow suffering from depression and nightmares, one of whose children had died from a heroin overdose. Aromatherapy massage using a blend of frankincense, bergamot, clary sage and jasmine gradually cured her of her nightmares and depression, and enabled her to give up her nightly sleeping pill.

* Penguin Books, 1998

Your aromatherapist may also suggest nutritional changes, or supplements, Bach Flower Remedies or herbal remedies to take at home.

A full aromatherapy treatment must be given by a professional but your therapist may make up a mixture of oils for use at home, perhaps to rub into painful joints or as a relaxant in the bath. Oils can also be inhaled, either by putting a drop or two on a handkerchief, or as an inhalation in boiling water.

You can buy essential oils in health food shops and pharmacies, and from herbalists; make sure they are reputable brands. Good quality oils include those made by Body Treats, Fleur, Neal's Yard Apothecary, Shirley Price and Robert Tisserand. Some shops make up their own cheaper brands which may be of inferior quality or heavily diluted; they smell nice but don't do much for you. Unfortunately, good oils can be expensive; prices vary according to the rarity of the plant. Blue Camomile, for instance, which is excellent for insomnia, costs around £18 for 5ml.

More moderately priced oils which are helpful for sleep are firstly lavender, which is extremely versatile; it's good for burns, insect bites, period problems and strengthening the immune system, among other properties. Neroli, marjoram, lemongrass, and linden (lime) blossom are all soothing; geranium helps to create balance and harmony; melissa oil is uplifting, and ylang-ylang will help lift depression. (Ylang-ylang also has a reputation as an aphrodisiac, so using it for a bedtime massage might not lead immediately to sleep.) Any of these oils can be used in the bath. To aid sleep, you can also put two or three drops on your pillow (but avoid direct skin contact) or on a handkerchief to sniff if you wake in the night.

If you have a partner or friend who will give your neck, shoulders and spine a gentle massage, you can make up your own massage oil. Use three or four drops of a single aromatherapy oil or two drops each of two oils in an egg-cup full of a base oil such as sweet almond or grape-seed.

If you make up larger amounts remember that once mixed, they will not retain their properties for very long. Keep the mixture in a dark, air-tight bottle and use it within three months. Don't use the same oil or oil mixture consecutively for too long, as it may lose its initial impact.

Caution: Essential oils are extremely potent, and should not be used neat on your skin; you could have an allergic reaction or, like the man who unwittingly used neat rosemary on his head for baldness, you could suffer from even more severe insomnia and 'mental chatter'.

Never take aromatherapy oils internally (unless prescribed by a medical aromatherapist).

BACH FLOWER REMEDIES

Bach Flower Remedies were the discovery of Dr Edward Bach (pronounced 'Batch', though a lot of people understandably pronounce it as they do the composer's name). A physician of Welsh descent, highly intuitive and sensitive, he spent his working life seeking ever purer methods of healing. After qualifying at University College Hospital he worked as a pathologist and bacteriologist, and then took up homoeopathy.

He came to the conclusion that illnesses are caused by negative mental states which, if prolonged, damage physical health. Conversely happiness, based on being in touch with one's higher self and life's purpose, allows the body to return to its natural state of good health.

In 1934 Dr Bach left his Harley Street practice to seek in the countryside plants that were appropriate to specific mental states. By holding his hand over plants to sense their energy, he intuitively discovered 38 remedies for different states of mind, testing them on himself and others.

He listed seven main moods: fear, uncertainty, lack of interest in the present, loneliness, over-sensitivity to influences, despair, and over-concern for others. He subdivided these, for example finding seven remedies for different kinds of fear including mimulus for fear of known causes, and aspen for fear of the unknown. He also created a thirty-ninth, Rescue Remedy, composed of five remedies, to be used for physical and mental shock, accidents and traumas.

There is no known scientific reason why these remedies should work, but the quantity of grateful letters received at the Bach Centre attests to the fact that they do. Without ever having advertised, the Centre is constantly busy, making and distributing the remedies, giving personal consultations and answering enquiries from all over the world.

Bach Remedies can be effective by themselves, and are an excellent adjunct to any other treatment you may be having. They can be made up in combinations of up to six remedies, since people often suffer from more than one symptom: some practitioners find it more effective to prescribe one at a time. Results can be instant or may take a few months; they occur so naturally that people sometimes only notice the change in themselves much later, looking back.

With their healing effect on mental states, the remedies can be very helpful with insomnia. Since they are chosen according to the personality, symptoms and attitudes of the sufferer, different remedies will suit different people. For example, for insomnia caused by a sudden bereavement, suitable remedies might include star of Bethlehem for shock, honeysuckle for a tendency to live in the past and perhaps chicory for self-pity. Willow is good for resentment, and holly for anger, olive for exhaustion of mind and body. A workaholic secretary who suffered from migraines as well as insomnia was prescribed oak for over-conscientiousness and olive for her exhaustion; after taking them for two months her migraines and insomnia had totally cleared up.

Bach Remedies can also help people coming off tranquillizers and sleeping pills by dealing with any old anxieties and worries that re-emerge during withdrawal.

HOMOEOPATHY

Homoeopathy is another complete system of medicine which can treat insomniacs on many levels, including the body, mind, and energy system. Developed during the eighteenth century by a German doctor, Samuel Hahnemann, it is based on giving minute doses of natural substances (plants, bee stings and so on) which, instead of suppressing symptoms, encourage the body to fight back.

The choice of remedies is based on the supposition that 'like cures like': if you give certain substances, for example quinine, to a healthy person, that person will develop the symptoms of a fever; therefore giving it to someone feverish will produce a cure. (Thus one of many possible remedies for insomnia is derived from caffeine.)

Over 20 years Hahnemann built up a complete repertoire of symptoms brought on by different remedies. He also experimented with making finer and finer dilutions of these remedies; at each stage of the dilution he subjected the solution to 'succussion'; banging it repeatedly on a hard surface to ensure the drops were thoroughly mixed. Without succussion, the remedies were ineffective, and it has continued to be an essential part of the process of making up homoeopathic medicines. Continuing with dilution and succussion, Hahnemann ended up with a finished product of so high a potency (i.e. highly diluted) that no molecules remained of the original substance.

It is this last fact that has made many scientists and medical doctors highly sceptical about homoeopathy, although its effectiveness has been shown time and again, both in individual patients and in some scientifically conducted trials. The reason why these highly diluted potencies work probably lies in the field of energy medicine, which is a very new area of exploration.

Whatever the scientific explanation, a number of medically trained doctors these days take further training in homoeopathy, which they find gentler and safer than many conventional drugs, and there are a few homoeopathic hospitals where you can be treated under the NHS. There are also numbers of non-medical homoeopaths who, while they have not gone through medical school, have usually taken a longer training in homoeopathy itself than qualified doctors. There used to be considerable friction between medical and non-medical practitioners, but these days the two groups are beginning to draw closer.

At the first consultation, the practitioner will ask the patient all kinds of questions: about his or her emotions, tastes in food, dreams, feelings and attitudes, and so on, as well as about any physical symptoms. The remedy or remedies will only be prescribed when a complete picture of the person has been built up.

The homoeopathic treatment of insomnia, says a homoeopath, 'is not something you can treat in isolation. You really do have to look at the whole person.' Since insomnia is often part of a whole conglomerate of symptoms, often going back to patterns developed in childhood or adolescence, or resulting from some later trauma, remedies will be chosen to deal both with the symptoms and their underlying causes.

For people coming off sleeping pills or other addictions homoeopathic remedies help to strengthen the system at the same time as clearing it. If during withdrawal people find themselves re-experiencing the emotional problems that caused them to become addicted in the first place, a good homoeopath will also supply reassurance and counselling, or refer patients for counselling if necessary.

Homoeopathy is excellent and safe for children and babies, who respond to it very well. Since the remedies take effect over time, there are some risks in trying to treat yourself long-term, but a child who swallows a bottle of homoeopathic tablets in one go is unlikely to come to any harm.

SELF-HELP

Although there are some homoeopathic sleeping pills on the market, they may not be suitable for everyone. The *Materia Medica*, the homoeopath's 'bible', includes many pages describing a vast range of types of insomnia ('racing thoughts', 'early waking', 'fear', 'anxiety', 'worse in morning' and so on) and specific remedies for each.

So it isn't possible to recommend a blanket remedy for everyone. A homoeopathic pharmacist may be willing to make up a remedy for you, but would probably advise you to consult a professional homoeopath as well.

KINESIOLOGY

Kinesiology is a way of examining and rebalancing the whole person. It can help the insomniac by identifying and correcting imbalances in body and mind, using a series of muscle tests and other techniques. It was the brainchild of an American chiropractor, Dr George Goodheart, who found that by testing the strength of specific muscles in a systematic way, it is possible to evaluate the patient's state as a whole: nutritional/chemical, emotional, musculo-skeletal and energetic.

Dr Goodheart called this system Applied Kinesiology. There are also simplified forms such as Touch for Health and Balanced Health, which are intended only for family use or as an adjunct to another therapy.

Some practitioners work purely as kinesiologists, while a number use kinesiology combined with other skills. An extremely basic form consists of testing whether a person's arm becomes weaker or stronger in reaction to certain foods, substances, or thoughts. This can look impressive; it is fascinating to see how an anxious thought, for instance, or a sugar-lump in the mouth, can cause someone's arm instantly to weaken, while a happy thought or a bite of an apple will strengthen it. However, serious kinesiologists regard this as a party trick: properly practised kinesiology is a great deal more complex.

It is based on the knowledge of a whole series of connections between particular muscles, organs, glands and bodily systems, including the acupuncture meridians and the circuitry of the brain and nervous system. So for correct treatment it's important to go to somebody who has done a reasonable amount of training, as well as being a good counsellor.

For insomnia, says kinesiologist Maggie La Tourelle: 'The first consideration would be to look for a balance in life, including nutrition, exercise and fresh air. Is the person in over-load or under-load? Some people don't sleep because they are not doing enough in their lives, and are not satisfied or motivated; if they're not expelling healthy energy during the day this can disturb them at night. Or are they working too hard? I would probably find all this out through counselling. I would look at the various stressors – emotional, work, environmental, chemical and so on, and identify where the stress is, both by counselling and by muscle testing.'

Muscle-testing is a way of asking the body non-verbal questions, to which its reactions give a truthful reply. To detect nutritional deficiencies and allergic reactions, the kinesiologist tests the strength of particular muscles in response to the patient's contact with items of food, vitamin and mineral samples and so on.

What is actually being tested is the brain's response to two things at once: holding the muscle in a particular position, together with another factor, like food. If there is a stress caused by the food, the brain cannot respond to the muscle test, and the muscle weakens. Items you need will strengthen the muscles, while items that are not therapeutic will weaken them. This is very useful if you are uncertain what supplements to take; Dr Goodheart once tested a film star who was taking 56 nutrients, and found she only needed four!

The kinesiologist can also 'ask' the body which of the various aspects – emotional, structural and so on – needs treating first, and whether any other treatment is needed. Once the areas of weakness have been discovered, he or she applies various techniques to strengthen and rebalance the body and its circuits. These include light massage on body reflexes to stimulate the lymphatic and vascular systems, and touching or holding the meridians and acupuncture points to release energy. Treatment includes nutritional and dietary advice;

the kinesiologist may also recommend Bach Flower Remedies.

An important aspect of kinesiology consists of techniques for creating balance in the brain, both between the left and right hemispheres, and also the forebrain (to do with future projects) and the back-brain (to do with memory and the past), which are often in conflict with each other. If the insomnia is caused by an over-stress on the logical hemisphere and neglect of the intuitive side, the balance is restored by using a number of brain integration techniques. One of these consists of drawing a large 'lazy 8' (the figure 8 lying on its side); then keeping your nose pointed towards the centre, follow the 8 round with your eyes for a minute or two. This can improve concentration and memory, among other benefits.

Another helpful technique, Emotional Stress Release, gently clears emotional trauma. By placing his or her hands on the patient's temples, the kinesiologist takes the charge out of an emotionally charged event, so that the memory is no longer disturbing. Clients can be taught to do this for themselves at home, which could be very helpful if a memory keeps you awake at night.

Kinesiologists may suggest other physical or mental exercises to do at home, including writing or repeating affirmations (positive statements), so that the balance can be maintained. 'I think that's very important,' says Maggie La Tourelle. 'So that people know they can leave the therapist's room and do something for themselves.'

MASSAGE

Massage is another helpful and enjoyable way of dealing with the stresses associated with insomnia, particularly for people who find it difficult to relax. To lie on a couch having your body caringly tended to can ease away all kinds of muscular and mental tensions. Touch and relaxation are healing in themselves; in addition, massage stimulates the circulation of blood and lymph, boosting the flow of oxygen and essential nutrients in the blood and also helping the body to free itself of waste toxins. This can be particularly beneficial for problems like rheumatism and arthritis.

It's interesting how massage has taken off over the last decade or so in Britain, since the British are not famous for appreciating the power of touch. Some men, in particular, seem to find it hard to understand that touch can be intimate and healing without having to lead to a sexual clinch, and in some areas massage is only slowly losing its erotic associations. Yet it is one of the most ancient and most natural forms of therapy, practised since ancient times in the East, and adopted by Ancient Greek physicians as a valid aspect of medicine. It is now beginning to come into its own in the West, and is regarded as a valid therapy by both natural practitioners and hospital nurses.

Everyone can benefit from massage, from the very young to the very old. Baby massage is becoming quite popular; gently stroking your baby all over is not only soothing but will help him or her to grow up with a good sense of self-acceptance. Old people can benefit greatly from touch, and are often starved of it – a lack that can certainly contribute to insomnia. In addition, massage with a good oil helps to keep the skin strong and supple.

There are various methods of massage; probably the best-known is Swedish Massage which uses a variety of techniques to relieve stress, encourage circulation, take the tension out of tight muscles and break down fat. Becoming popular today is Intuitive Massage, which is less rigidly structured and also takes into account the body's energy system.

A professional massage can take an hour or longer, and is a very pleasant experience. These days massage therapists often use aromatherapy oils in their massage oils.

Self-help

Many people find that giving a massage is as soothing as receiving one; more than one massage therapist has told me that focusing their attention on the other person is like a form of meditation. Couples attending massage courses find that it brings them closer; non-sexual touch can have a loving quality that can feed back into your sex life. And for couples going through a bad patch, emotionally or sexually, learning massage together can sometimes break through barriers that talking can't.

Anyone can give a massage to their child, partner or relative, particularly concentrating on the neck and shoulders; but if you are untrained, keep your touch gentle – particularly if you massage someone's head. It's even nicer if you use a pleasantly scented aromatherapy oil. If you want to take it further, look out for evening classes or weekend courses. You can learn a great deal from books such as Lucinda Lidett's well-illustrated *Book of Massage* which gives instructions for intuitive massage, shiatsu and reflexology, with sections on massaging babies and old people, and on the energy system and centres.

MASSAGING THE FEET

This can also be extraordinarily soothing, mentally and physically; among other benefits it draws tension away from the head, helping to calm an over-active mind. If you have a partner who is willing to massage your feet, try it after getting into bed; you may well find yourself drifting off to sleep.

Foot massage is also a very good way to get a fractious baby to settle down – just gently stroke the feet for a few minutes after a bath. Of course, with babies, you can do this at any time of day.

MASSAGING YOURSELF

Self-massage is obviously not as satisfactory as having someone doing it for you, but it can still be quite soothing. Starting with your head, go down whatever bits of you you can reach, gently pressing and releasing with your palms and fingers. Then use your hands to lightly brush yourself down, smoothing out the energy field around you.

Simply massaging your hands and fingers can also release quite a lot of tension. Try it: you may find yourself yawning.

MEDICAL HERBALISM

Herbal medicine has been used by mankind throughout the ages and all over the world, and is growing in popularity today in response to concern about drugs, and the desire for more natural forms of medication. Herbalists, like any other natural practitioners, feel that relying on herbs simply as tranquillizers is much the same as relying on medical drugs unless you also deal with the causes of your insomnia. The herbalist's aim is not merely to treat symptoms, but to prescribe medicines that will improve general vitality, clear the system of toxins, and restore balance and harmony; good sleep then comes about naturally.

Many modern drugs are based on plants: aspirin is extracted from willow, and digitalis from the foxglove, for instance. What modern science has done is to isolate from these plants, the 'active ingredient' that provides relief or cure. What it has overlooked in this process is that each herb contains a *balance* of ingredients which counteract any side effects from the active ingredient taken in isolation. They also contain health-promoting vitamins and trace elements. Herbalism is therefore generally very safe and properly prescribed medicines have no side-effects. It is true, of course, that some herbs are harmful, and you should go to a qualified medical herbalist.

Herbalists treat much the same range of problems as GPs, and their diagnostic techniques resemble those of medical doctors, using the same equipment for testing blood pressure and so on. As well as assessing symptoms, practitioners evaluate the overall balance of the body's various systems to ascertain underlying disharmonies, and they prescribe on the basis of the whole person rather than symptoms alone. Therefore, as with homoeopathy and other natural medicines, prescriptions for the same disease will vary for individual patients. Different herbs would be appropriate, for instance, for sleeplessness caused by anxiety, digestive problems, hormonal imbalance, and so on.

For insomnia, the herbalist would want to find out what is contributing to lack of sleep. Practitioners look into the patient's lifestyle, including exercise and nutrition, and will recommend a healthy, wholefood diet; treatment is regarded as a co-operative effort in which patients play their part by making any changes that are indicated.

Medicines are usually dispensed in liquid form as tinctures. Herbal medicine can act quite fast, particularly when patients pay attention to a good diet. In chronic cases, however, it can take time to restore health as the medicines work gently and thoroughly, both detoxifying the patient's system and building up his or her strength.

Self-help

Herbal medicines can be useful to try out at home for minor health problems in adults and children, and you can learn to use them from a number of books. If you take a herbal remedy for a chronic condition, you can expect some improvement within two or three days, but it may take two or more weeks to get the full effect. So take any remedy for a month to give it a fair trial, and when you do improve, taper off gradually. Herbs are not truly addictive, but since they act upon the central nervous system they should not be taken regularly for weeks on end.

NATUROPATHY

Naturopaths not only advise on nutrition but look at their patients' whole lifestyle, including their working life and any anxieties causing particular stress, and will work with patients to deal with the problems underlying insomnia. Many naturopaths are also trained in osteopathy (described in the next section), which helps to relieve structural and muscular tensions and pain.

Sometimes called nature cure, naturopathy is one of the best established forms of natural and holistic medicine; it has had its followers in Britain since well before the Second World War. It is based on the principle that the body has its own restorative powers, and under the right conditions will heal itself. The right conditions for good health include nutrition, exercise, relaxation, a balanced and unstressed musculo-skeletal system, and a positive outlook on life. Treatment therefore consists chiefly of removing impediments to health rather than adding extras, although naturopaths may use some herbal and homoeopathic preparations as well as nutritional supplements when appropriate to individual needs.

Practitioners may advocate fasting, to rid the body of accumulated poisons – either a complete fast, or a few days on fruit or fruit juices. Fasting doesn't suit everyone, and the naturopath will take your personal needs and system into account before recommending it. Hydrotherapy (water cure) is also traditionally associated with naturopathy, including treatments such as encouraging the circulation around arthritic joints by alternate applications of hot and cold water, or using sitz baths to improve the circulation in the abdominal area. More elaborate forms of hydrotherapy are applied at some health farms.

Naturopaths will also advise on appropriate exercise and relaxation techniques, and support you in making changes to your lifestyle.

OSTEOPATHY AND CHIROPRACTIC

Manipulative techniques can often help insomniacs, and not only by relieving pain in the back or other joints; treatment can be an excellent stress reliever. Insomnia, headaches, migraines and general tension are, for example, often caused or exacerbated by problems in the vertebrae of the neck, which both the osteopath and the chiropractor can relieve or cure.

Both these methods of treating the musculo-skeletal system (the bones, muscles and joints) are becoming increasingly accepted by orthodox medicine. The two therapies were evolved independently in America towards the end of the nineteenth century, and there are variations between them, although some techniques are common to both. There are also variations between the techniques used by practitioners from different training schools (particularly the British Chiropractic Association and the McTimoney Chiropractic Association with its 'whole-body' approach.)

Both osteopathy and chiropractic are based on the principle that the health of the spine has a profound effect on overall well-being. The spinal cord is an extension of the brain, and connects with all the organs of the body via the circulatory and nervous systems. So although people generally seek these therapies for back and joint pain, they can be beneficial for a wide range of problems as diverse as asthma, migraine, indigestion, hiatus hernia, pre-menstrual tension and so on. Some practitioners are good counsellors; some also take a particular interest in nutrition, and can advise you on diet and supplements, particularly those who have also trained in naturopathy.

Adjusting the vertebrae is not usually painful, and the effects can be extremely relaxing. One woman who had barely slept for four years after injuring her neck in a car accident eventually visited a chiropractor; after treatment she fell asleep for several hours, and subsequently returned to a normal sleep pattern.

Nowadays quite elderly people are turning to these therapies for help with arthritic and back pain with good results. Manipulation may not cure the arthritis, but it can relieve the pressure on arthritic joints and improve the circulation of blood around them, helping to remove toxic waste. Practitioners have a variety of techniques at their disposal, as well as, or instead of, actual manipulation which might be over-traumatic for the old or those in very severe pain. Soft tissue techniques (specific ways of massaging the muscles) also help to realign joints, relax over-tense bodies, and boost the circulation of blood and lymphatic drainage.

A woman in her forties went to an osteopath specifically for her insomnia; for about a year she had been waking at three in the morning, only falling asleep again when it was nearly time to get up. She was not under any special stress, but was overweight and suffered from indigestion. The osteopath first treated her for muscle tension and restriction in the shoulder girdle; in the next two months, as these tensions relaxed, she began to return to normal sleep.

CRANIAL OSTEOPATHY AND CRANIO-SACRAL THERAPY

This is an extremely gentle approach to manipulation practised by some osteopaths and chiropractors as well as cranio-sacral therapists. It is based on the connection between the cranium (the skull) and the sacrum, the shield-shaped bone at the base of the spine.

Practitioners often work simply by placing a hand gently on the relevant parts of the spine, relieving tension and encouraging the flow of cerebro-spinal fluid, which nourishes the spinal cord. This is extremely relaxing in itself, as well as curative. They may also treat the skull and jaw, often an area of much tension.

Cranial treatment can be very helpful for both babies and mothers after a difficult birth. A cranial check-up after birth might prevent a lot of 'inexplicable' problems in babies.

A number of cranio-sacral practitioners are very intuitive, and can tune into the emotional origins of their patients' pain, helping to heal mind and body simultaneously.

REFLEXOLOGY AND REFLEX ZONE THERAPY

'In the vast majority of the people I treat,' says a former nurse turned reflexologist, 'by the time I get to the second foot, their heads are nodding.' Reflexology is yet another complementary therapy that provides deep relaxation as well as therapeutic treatment for a number of ailments. Its origins are very old: an Ancient Egyptian wall painting shows two people having their feet treated. Reflexology was rediscovered in the 1920s by an American physician Dr William Fitzgerald, and is growing in popularity today.

Like acupuncture, it is based on the theory that there are channels of energy flowing through the body. These channels are not identical, yet both therapies are effective – which is one of those mysteries of alternative medicine. In the case of reflexology, there are ten channels, which can be tapped into through specific reflex zones in the feet and hands. The feet themselves represent a kind of map of the body, with the big toes relating to the head and neck, and the bony side of the foot to the spine; reflex points for the liver, kidneys and other organs are found in the soft part of the arch, and so on.

Reflexologists are trained to sense energy blockages in the feet, and massage techniques to unblock them, stimulating the energy flow, and encouraging the body to heal itself. Some patients can actually sense the energy in the part of the body relating to the point on the foot being treated; it can feel like a mild electric shock.

You may be treated sitting up or lying down. The practitioner will give a complete treatment to both feet, and then focus on any problem areas. For insomnia, particular attention is likely to be given to the head area, including the pituitary gland (the master gland of the hormonal system) and to the adrenals, which may be overworked by stress. The solar plexus (about a third of the way down the sole of the foot) is another point that is likely to receive extra attention, and you may be asked to breathe deeply while it is being treated; this is excellent for stress.

Reflexology is particularly good for conditions involving congestion – sinusitis, migraine, asthma, a sluggish liver, fluid retention and so on. Sometimes people treated for such conditions experience a reaction as their bodies throw out toxins, possibly in the form of vomiting or diarrhoea, after which they feel very much better and clearer.

Reflexology is also good for releasing emotional congestion, especially when the therapist is receptive and a good counsellor. The reflexologist quoted in the first paragraph treated a woman who had been sleeping badly and feeling generally stressed since the recent death of her mother. During her mother's illness she had held back her emotions in order to be 'strong for the family'. After two treatments she found herself in floods of tears; the reflexologist reassured her that this was absolutely right and healthy: there had been an emotional build-up which needed to be released. The client understood the sense of this; following this episode she slept much better.

On the whole, treatment is fairly painless; now and again pressure on a particular site of trouble can hurt, but this does not last. Reflexology is in fact very good for the relief of chronic pain, possibly more effective than drugs and without the side effects. It is also helpful for hormonal imbalances and a variety of problems that may be affecting your sleep; after a treatment most people sleep extra well. As with other natural therapies, a course of several treatments will be needed to bring about a lasting effect, and patients can help themselves by following their practitioner's recommendations about diet and so on.

Reflex Zone Therapy, which works along very similar lines, is taught to and practised by qualified nurses and physiotherapists. Used in a maternity unit, it has been found particularly beneficial for post-birth problems, such as wind, and difficulty in passing urine. One new mother who was suffering from tension because of domestic problems asked for a sleeping tablet; since she needed to wake easily should her child need attention during the night, she was offered Reflex Zone Therapy instead. She was asleep before the treatment was complete, and woke six hours later to feed her baby.*

* Margarita Evans, 'Reflex Zone Therapy for Mothers', *Nursing Times*, (24–30 January 1990)

SHIATSU

Shiatsu, also called acupressure, is a form of oriental massage developed in Japan at the beginning of the twentieth century. It is based on the same principles as acupuncture, but uses the hands, fingers, knuckles and even elbows to stimulate the acupuncture points and rebalance the meridians. Practitioners also use the breath, breathing from the *hara*, the energy centre in the abdominal area, to direct energy into their hands.

Like acupuncture, Shiatsu helps to rebalance the body's energy system, relieving aches and pains, tension and stress. Ideally it is used to maintain health and vitality, rather than for curing disease, although in Japan, when practised by experienced practitioners, it can be as effective as acupuncture and medical herbalism.

A shiatsu practitioner may show you how to self-massage
the points that will help you relax and improve your sleep.
If you have someone to practise with, you can learn some
self-help techniques from books, but if you have a medical
condition, do not use it as a substitute for proper
treatment. There is a form of self-shiatsu called Do-In;
look out for evening classes or weekend workshops.

SPIRITUAL HEALING

Spiritual healing, with its calming and uplifting effects on
mind and body, can be extremely helpful with insomnia.
It is also compatible with any other treatment you may be
having, whether physical or psychological.

A healing session can last from 20 minutes to an hour.
The healer will usually chat with you first, and then ask
you to sit or lie down; you don't have to remove any
clothing. Many of them work almost purely in the energy

field around the body, in which they can sense areas where there are problems. Others will lay their hands directly on painful areas, often relieving pain very rapidly. Many combine the two techniques.

Healing is usually a very relaxing experience; some people go to sleep during a session, and many sleep extra well afterwards. Patients often leave feeling emotionally and spiritually uplifted. Healers can also provide regular support for people going through difficult times, and help them to build up their own inner resources. Sometimes during a healing session patients find themselves crying, releasing pent-up stress or grief.

Many healers have clairvoyant or strongly intuitive gifts, which can help them to pinpoint the causes of people's problems. Many, too, are excellent intuitive counsellors, and healer training courses increasingly emphasize the development of counselling skills. It is important, they say, to heal not only the physical but the emotional/spiritual causes of illness. A number of them encourage patients to take part in the release of past stresses, through visualization, meditation, and forgiveness.

One woman began seeing a healer specifically for her insomnia, which had been extremely severe for several years; she was only sleeping for two or three hours a night. She had a number of emotional problems and, having decided to sort herself out, was also seeing a psychotherapist. Initially she found herself sleeping much better for two or three nights following each weekly healing session; as time went on, these two or three nights extended into seven nights a week.

Also available …

The Energy Technique

Simple secrets for a lifetime of vitality and energy

VERA PEIFFER

Are you feeling exhausted and wiped out? Do you need to recharge your batteries?

Packed with simple, fun and effective techniques, this little book will leave you refreshed, revitalized and raring to go!